Naturopathy in South India

Sir Henry Wellcome Asian Series

Edited by

Dominik Wujastyk
Paul U. Unschuld
Charles Burnett

Editorial Board

Donald J. Harper
Ch. Z. Minkowski
Guy Attewell
Nikolaj Serikoff

VOLUME 17

The titles published in this series are listed at *brill.com/was*

Naturopathy in South India

Clinics between Professionalization and Empowerment

By

Eva Jansen

BRILL

LEIDEN | BOSTON

Cover illustration: Naturopathic patient taking a full mud bath in the UGLA Ashram. PHOTO TAKEN BY THE AUTHOR.

Library of Congress Cataloging-in-Publication Data

Names: Jansen, Eva, author.
Title: Naturopathy in South India : clinics between professionalization and
   empowerment / by Eva Jansen.
Description: Leiden : Boston : Brill, [2016] | Series: Sir Henry Wellcome
   Asian series ; 17 | Includes bibliographical references and index.
Identifiers: LCCN 2016023232 (print) | LCCN 2016026597 (ebook) | ISBN
   9789004324848 (hardback : alk. paper) | ISBN 9789004325104 (ebook) | ISBN
   9789004325104 (E-book)
Subjects: LCSH: Naturopathy--South India. | Herbs--Therapeutic use--South
   India.
Classification: LCC RZ440 .J36 2016 (print) | LCC RZ440 (ebook) | DDC
   615.5/35--dc23
LC record available at https://lccn.loc.gov/2016023232

Want or need Open Access? Brill Open offers you the choice to make your research freely accessible online in exchange for a publication charge. Review your various options on brill.com/brill-open.

Typeface for the Latin, Greek, and Cyrillic scripts: "Brill". See and download: brill.com/brill-typeface.

ISSN 1570-1484
ISBN 978-90-04-32484-8 (hardback)
ISBN 978-90-04-32510-4 (e-book)

To Ravi

∵

Contents

Acknowledgments

In order to write *Naturopathy in South India: Clinics between Professionalization and Empowerment*, I required the assistance of quite a few people and I would like to take the opportunity to thank them all for their contributions.

First, I would like to thank Claudia Lang, who gave me the chance to participate in her research project and supported me over the years in writing and publishing on the topic of Naturopathy. She commented on almost every stage of my work and guided me through the resolution of many theoretical dilemmas. During the time that we worked together, we not only shared literature and ideas, but we also became friends.

I would also like to thank my doctoral supervisor, Frank Heidemann, who provided valuable suggestions on this project and even visited us at our home in Kerala. Gabriele Alex, my second supervisor, also displayed great interest in my work.

Quite a number of anthropologists contributed through conversations, talks and suggestions, including Mireille Mazard, Hans-Jörg Dilger, Christoph Cyranski, Nasima Selim, Heide Castañeda and the rest of the AG Medical Anthropology network. Their regular meetings helped me to structure the doctoral thesis on which this book is based and to keep me focused.

Thanks to Josephine Horlor and Karen Dyer who did a great job with language editing and commenting on the manuscript. Stefan Krovinovic and Hugo Hertz also contributed to this book by helping me to display pictures and figures throughout the chapters.

For all the practitioners who recognize themselves either directly or indirectly in these pages, I would like to express my deepest gratitude for their friendliness, time and patience. A special thanks goes to Dr. Baby's family, who always graciously welcomed me into their home. I owe this introduction to Murphy Halliburton, and it was most valuable to me.

Additionally, I would like to thank Dr. Vadakkanchery and his wife Soumnya; Dr. Madhavan from the MNCC in Bakkalam; Father Thomas Maliekal in Ernakulam; Dr. Jyotsna and Kalyan Ulpalakshan from the GNH in Thrissur; Dr. Balakrishnan Nair from the NLH in Kozhikode; Dr. Savitha from Bangalore; Dr. Naveen and Dr. Ashok Kumar Sharma from NIMHANS, also in Bangalore; Dr. Babu Joseph and Dr. Sathyanath from NIN in Pune; Father Philip Neru in Trivandrum; Dr. Nalvazhvu from the UGLA in Shivasailam; Dr. Ashraf Kalayam in Kozhikode; Surender Sandhu from the CCRYN in Delhi; Mr. Kurian from Kottayam, and Dr. S. K. Madhavan and his colleagues from the MNCC, who all devoted much time and energy to answering my questions and sharing the secrets of Naturopathy with me. Throughout the rest of the text, all of these practitioners are referred to by the names they used in our introduction. With two exceptions I did not use pseudonyms for the practitioners since all of them had an interest in disseminating their knowledge in their own names.

I would like to thank Sanat and Babu Appad, who helped me with translations, explanations and also with traveling, especially in the first year of my research. Sanat continues to answer my questions via email and on Facebook and keeps me up-to-date on the naturopathic scene in Kerala. A significant contribution was made by Indu P, a graduate student of English literature from Kozhikode University, who translated many books, articles and speeches for me with great patience and incredible reliability and also continues to answer my questions over email. During my fieldwork, I became friends with Xavier Manickathan, Soni Somarajan, Sajo George, Sobi Devadasan, Sister Tessy, Kiran Jonnalagadda, Zainab Bawa and many others who continuously supported me by offering explanations about aspects of India, Kerala and Naturopathy that had otherwise left me confused.

Many patients generously contributed to this book by telling their own very personal stories. As I wanted to keep all of their names anonymous, I would like to offer a general, heartfelt thanks to all those who recognize themselves in this book, and to all the others who have shared their suffering and hopes with me, especially "Mrs. Marple." For patients I decided to use pseudonyms only.

I am indebted to my hosts in Kottakkal, Kerala – Babu, Ancy and their wonderful children Jovitha and Adina – for their very personal support. They treated me like a full member of the family and continually answered my questions about medicine, health, language and culture in Kerala. I spent many months in their home and always felt very welcomed and relaxed.

The first two years of my study were funded by the DFG (the Deutsche Forschungsgemeinschaft). Together with Claudia Lang, I worked on the project *Glocalizing Depression in Kerala*. Thanks also goes to the DAAD (Deutscher Akademischer Austauschdienst), who sponsored my journey to the *American Anthropological Association Annual Meeting* in 2011 in Montreal, Canada to present portions of this work.

I would like to thank Dr. Ohlert and his fantastic team in the Sebastianeum in Bad Wörishofen. In particular, the comment by Mr. Bohmhammel, a physiotherapist, on the effectiveness of the treatments through "*picking up the patient*" was very convincing to me.

The anonymous reviewer of this book at Brill helped me to organize my thoughts and to more clearly shape my arguments. I want to thank him or her for reading the manuscript very carefully and providing useful, constructive comments that contributed significantly to this work.

Writing this book, and actually finishing it, proved not to be an easy task. The daily routine of writing in a desolate corner was quite hard to bear, especially since my first child was born during the process of rewriting. Keeping this in mind, tremendous thanks go to close friends and family – my father, my mother, her husband and my brother – who have given me unwavering encouragement and support over the years.

The last person I want to thank listened to my challenges, proceedings and arguments over and over: my husband. He made a great effort supporting me through endless talks at any time of the day about Naturopathy and – most important – he provided me with tremendous encouragement to finish my book in a timely manner.

List of Illustrations

Figures

Tables

Map

Abbreviations

AINCF	All India Nature Cure Federation, Delhi
AYUSH	A ministry of the Indian government that supports non-allopathic medical systems such as Ayurveda, Yoga and Naturopathy, Unani, Siddha, Homeopathy and most recently Sowa-Rigpa
BNYS	Bachelor of Naturopathy and Yogic Science
CCRYN	Central Council for Research in Yoga and Naturopathy, Delhi
DNYT	Diploma of Naturopathic and Yogic Therapy, an alternative degree in Naturopathy and Yoga
GNH	Gandhiji Naturopathy Hospital, Thrissur
INYGMA	Indian Naturopathy and Yoga Graduate Medical Association
ISM	Indian Systems of Medicine, Thiruvananthapuram
MDNIY	Morarji Desai National Institute of Yoga, Delhi
MNCC	Mahatma Gandhi Nature Cure Center, located near Thalassery
NIMHANS	National Institute of Mental Health and Neurosciences, Bangalore
NIN	National Institute of Naturopathy, Pune
NLH	Nature Life Hospital, Kozhikode
PG	Postgraduate
UGLA	Universal Good Life Ashram, Sivasailam

PART 1

Naturopathy in Theory

∵

Introduction to Part 1

The increasing multiplicity of medical options in many places of the world affected by globalization can lead to a pervasive insecurity among those seeking care about whether the chosen medical treatment is the right one. This confusion is heightened when even within the same medical system there are points of disagreement concerning the "right" treatment option and even the etiology of the ailment. Patients may ask themselves: does this option fight my ailment quickly? Does it produce side effects that need further treatment? Am I able to integrate the treatment easily into my lifestyle? Is the treatment pleasant and enjoyable, or is it painful? Is my quality of life maintained? Will the treatment prolong my life? Is the treatment reproducible and transparent to me? Do I trust the practitioner because she or he takes enough time and shows enough empathy to explain what is wrong with me?

Naturopathy offers relatively simple answers to all of these questions. It can be easily explained, understood and implemented. In the hyper-globalized and complex 21st century health care market, Naturopathy's simplicity is one reason it attracts increasing numbers of health-seekers worldwide suffering from a wide variety of ailments.

Naturopathy is an eclectic healing system with its roots in 19th century Europe and USA. Although nowadays its ideology and healing methods are quite heterogeneous and have spread to many parts of the world, all practitioners and activists identifying with Naturopathy share common ideological elements. The unifying principle underlying the heterogeneous forms of Naturopathy is a general critique of allopathic[1] practices, such as invasive surgical interventions and medication causing serious biochemical reactions as well as short- and long-term effects on the body. Supporters of Naturopathy believe that the body has its own healing power that can be activated by minimizing intake of harmful substances, and there is a great emphasis on education, prevention and client responsibility (Kirchfeld and Boyle 1994, Wendel 1951, Baer 2001, 2009). Furthermore, Naturopaths critique Allopathy as being rooted in capitalist principles such as efficacy, marketing, lobbying and an economy of time. This is the reason why a rejection of imperialistic, capitalist, non-humanitarian and neo-colonialist politics often is an integral element of Naturopathy. *Naturopathy in South India: Clinics between Professionalization and Empowerment* explores the Indian appropriation of Naturopathy.

---

1   The term Allopathy, first used by the founder of Homeopathy Samuel Hahnemann, describes a system that treats with oppositional medicine. I employ the term in this book because most of my informants used it. Alternatively, they also used "Western medicine," "biomedicine," "modern medicine," or "English medicine."

© KONINKLIJKE BRILL NV, LEIDEN, 2016 | DOI 10.1163/9789004325104_002

CHAPTER 1

Ambiguities: From the Evil in Baby Oil to Yogic Randomized Controlled Trials

I met Dr. Vadakkanchery for the first time during a naturopathic health camp in Chelembra, close to the University of Kozhikode in northern Kerala. This event gathered approximately 100 people together for three days in order to learn the *"naturopathic way of life."* In between teaching sessions, songs and quiz games, participants were served raw fruits or dried rice with raw vegetables. Most of the attendees lived in the surrounding area and suffered from conditions such as asthma, obesity, and allergies or even more serious diseases such as cancer or HIV. Most of them had previously sought healing from practitioners of several different medical systems, such as Allopathy, Homeopathy, Ayurveda, or religious healing. However, none had been successful. Thus, by visiting this naturopathic camp, they hoped to harness the curing power of nature.

Over the course of the first day, Dr. Vadakkanchery delivered several speeches on natural living and its implications. He explained that the cause of disease is *"toxification"* through the consumption of unnatural foods and products, Western influences and unhealthy lifestyles. In order to illustrate his arguments, Dr. Vadakkanchery held up a bottle of Johnson's Baby Oil, read the list of ingredients and stated that most of them are unclear, chemical and poisonous. When he arrived at the warning label at the bottom of the bottle – *"Keep out of reach of children"* – the crowd started to hoot. Later that day, Dr. Vadakkanchery introduced the first female speaker, who had given birth to her child in a *"natural way,"* meaning without the assistance of allopathic practitioners or treatments. This woman recounted her birth experience in the hospital where she had eaten only raw food. She rotated her healthy child repeatedly through the air and the crowd acknowledged her with enthusiastic applause. Attendees punctuated the session by asking questions and telling stories from their own lives. Children ran through the crowd and played noisily with each other next to the audience.

A speaker named Hira Ratan Manek had been invited to this event. He had become famous for living on sunlight only, without any kind of food or even liquid; this, according to Babu, my research assistant at the time, had been *"prove[n] by modern medical science and NASA."* Babu had even picked up his wife from work to give her the chance to see and hear the famous visitor. He was not the only one for whom the health camp offered a pleasing diversion from daily routines.

The health camp we were attending took place at a hospital of the Nature Life Group and was organized by the hospital administration. Dr. Vadakkanchery and his followers hoped to attract many visitors who would thereafter be ready to join one of the Nature Life Hospitals and, accordingly, have their diseases cured through a life lived more closely in tune with nature. Dr. Vadakkanchery does not hold a university medical degree; instead, he is trained as a social worker.

On another occasion about two months later, I was in Bangalore at the famous psychiatric hospital of NIMHANS for a conference entitled "*Yoga Therapies for Psychiatric Disorders.*" This conference was one of many on Naturopathy and Yoga in Bangalore and was organized by the Morarji Desai National Institute for Yoga in Delhi. In six sessions, presenters discussed the influence of Yoga and Naturopathy on current psychiatric diseases such as geriatric disorders, child disorders, depression, neurotic disorders and psychotic disorders. All of the roughly 80 participants in attendance were members of different university faculties, either of NIMHANS itself, an affiliated Yoga university, or a nearby naturopathic university in Mysore. The speakers, some of whom were about to finish their PhD degrees and others who were already employed as hospital-based practitioners, discussed the results of their studies on patients following naturopathic diets, treatment and Yoga practice. These studies had titles such as "*The Effect of Yoga and Naturopathy Therapy on Anxiety, Depression and Quality-of-Life among Caregivers of In-Patients with Neurological Disorders at a Tertiary Care Center in India: A Randomized Controlled Trial.*" The conference included an official introduction by the chairman of the Yoga Institute in Delhi, and a fixed time frame for questions and discussion after every session. On this occasion, I met a young PhD scholar from the affiliated Yoga university, Mr. Bose, who was investigating the effects of Naturopathy and Yoga on psychiatric diseases, primarily depression. In a subsequent interview, Mr. Bose explained his approach to and method of research. According to him, he had adopted a simple sampling method in which sixty participants were randomized into either a control or experimental group. Mr. Bose then assessed the participants' anxiety and depression levels with the Hospital Anxiety and Depression Scale (HADS), and their quality-of-life using a WHO-developed scale. Mr. Bose provided the experimental group with a structured Yoga and Naturopathy 10-day training module, which they continued to follow independently for an additional month. The control group, however, did not receive such training. In the end, both groups were reassessed using the same scales. The result, as Mr. Bose emphasizes, was a statistically significant decrease in anxiety and depression and improved quality-of-life among the subjects in the experimental group. Mr. Bose used a pen and paper to illustrate the $p<0.001$ significance level of the decrease, so that the impressive result would be as clear and convincing to me as possible.

At the end of our interview, Mr. Bose was not quite sure if his approach to Naturopathy had been thoroughly understood. I was already on my way out of the room, carrying my tape recorder and notebook, when he called me back in and asked me to sit down and switch on my recorder again. Then he continued:

> Naturopathy is not only a medical system, it is lifestyle modification. What we are doing currently is that we are going away from nature. That is why we are getting a lot of problems. We can do so many things scientifically, one day we might be able to go to the sun. So we should lead a lifestyle that is natural, not like getting medication, going with all the technology. Even I am a perfect full-time Naturopath. These principles persuaded me.

These divergent experiences with two people who both call themselves doctors of Naturopathy, Dr. Vadakkanchery and Mr. Bose, were initially quite confusing to me. Although ultimately both preached the same principles, their implementation of these principles differed significantly. At the same time, however, the dividing lines between personal conviction, lifestyle, method, scientific approach, self-representation, diffusion of knowledge and the way of legitimation seemed to blur, at times completely dissolving, in ways that will be described throughout the rest of these chapters.

This book is about the heterogeneity of socio-medical naturopathic practices in South India, principally in northern Kerala but also in the surrounding area. My aim is to analyze the specific historical and socio-cultural conditions in which Naturopathy evolved and became as popular as it is in South India today. Furthermore, I will examine the genesis of the dichotomy of practices and their relationship with one another: one approach that is rather informal and triggered by a critique of globalization, such as that espoused by Dr. Vadakkanchery, and another approach that aspires to be strictly evidence-based and fully professionalized, such as that practiced by Mr. Bose. What does this dichotomy, with its different underlying principles, mean for the actual treatment procedures used in hospitals? How do naturopathic agents appear in this scenario? What is the role of patients' choice and agency in the field of Naturopathy? These are the questions to which this book will be dedicated.

1   Floating Through Time and Across Space: Naturopathic Theories
         and Practices

Today, naturopathic theories and practices are widely known throughout the
world. However, as Dr. Vadakkanchery and Mr. Bose have demonstrated, these
practices can differ substantially both within the same location and across
locations. In order to clarify the relationship between the overall concept of
Naturopathy and its local variations, in the following section I will theoretically contextualize the field's basic assumptions.

Referring to the globalization theorist Appadurai, I use the term "*imagined
naturopathic worlds*" to reference local variations of Naturopathy (2002, 1996,
see also Hörbst and Krause 2004). Employing the concept of imagined worlds,
multiple contexts of Naturopathy are distributed worldwide via the histori-
cally-based imaginations of individuals or groups. Naturopathic assumptions
have been detached from their original locality and appropriated in multiple
new contexts of action. The original locality can be cited as the naturopathic
health movement of the 19th century, which took place primarily in central
Europe and to a much smaller extent in the U.S.

The unraveling of "scapes" is a productive technique to conceptualize imagined naturopathic worlds. Appadurai introduced five dimensions of scapes:
ethnoscapes, mediascapes, technoscapes, financescapes and ideoscapes. He
makes use of these scapes to describe dynamic flows and processes of globalization. In this context multiple possible actors can be identified, such as
religious communities, subcultures, and migrant groups, as well as material
products, concepts and ideas. An important factor is that these scapes are
never received passively but are always reinterpreted and appropriated in the
specific local context. As a continuation of this approach that situates it within
a medical context, Hörbst and Wolf (2003, 2014, see also Hörbst and Krause
2004) introduced the term medicoscapes:

> With reference to Appadurai, we understand this to mean globally dis-
> tributed scapes of people and organizations in the medicine sector which
> can be clustered locally but which can also connect places, people and
> organizations located far apart. These include people seeking and offer-
> ing international therapy, globally operating pharmaceutical firms, the
> WHO as the global biomedicine watchdog, organizations of so-called tra-
> ditional healers, regional non-medical practices and their adoption at
> other places, globally available forms of therapy and organizations con-
> ducting international development work in medical sectors (Hörbst and
> Wolf 2003: 4, translated by the author).

The worldwide phenomenon of Naturopathy is therefore best understood as a medicoscape: it constitutes a global landscape, consisting of uneven units and divergent, more-or-less intense elements that vary locally depending on the specificity of the particular place. An integral part of this theoretical concept is the possibility of construction, deconstruction and dynamic movement. Since the 19th century, multiple naturopathic concepts have been transferred to India from abroad and have subsequently been reshaped in the Indian context. The sociologist Robertson (1992) re-introduced the term glocalisation in order to define the relations and co-existence of multidimensional processes of globalization and their local and regional impacts and appropriations.

Naturopathy is a global concept, an imagined world with ongoing flows and circulations and diverse local appropriations. However, the present research on naturopathic practices in a locally-bound area shows the integration and transformation of ideas and aspects at the micro level. In India, Naturopathy is next to the imagined world an institutionalized medical system, delineated in theory and practice from other medical epistemologies.

2   Medical Pluralism and Epistemologies

The term "medical pluralism" was originally intended to describe multiple options for health care. It is clearly no coincidence that the term, first introduced by the anthropologist Charles Leslie in the 1970s, referred to medical systems in Asia. Anthropologists seemed to uncover the broadest spectrum of medical practices on that continent.

Leslie's two most significant works, *Asian Medical Systems* in 1976 and *Paths to Asian Medical Knowledge* (co-edited with Allan Young in 1992) have established a sound basis for researching medical systems and practices in various Asian countries. In these volumes, anthropologists aimed to do away with the assumption that patients all over the world rely solely on Allopathy. They examined medical traditions that were not subsumed under its dominant models, theories and practices, mainly in so-called Third World countries.

Although some articles in Leslie's volume did analyze flows and linkages between the systems, the first anthology creates the impression that the systems described are mostly self-contained and well-delineated. In the second volume in 1992, Leslie divided Asian medicine into three sectors: Chinese medicine, Ayurveda and Islamic humoral traditions. He contrasted Allopathy as a fourth medical system. This fragmentation of Asian practices into four systems has since been revised, as modern research has identified a much more complex composition of medical practices.

In 1980, Arthur Kleinman, one of the pioneers of medical anthropology, described a structural model that can be applied to homogenous, post-traditional societies. In this model, health care consists of the popular, professional, and folk sectors. According to Kleinman, the popular sector encompasses treatment by non-professionals, such as oneself, members of the family, or the wider community. This applies to most health care and is therefore the largest sector and also the link between all the systems. The professional sector in most societies is simply allopathic medicine. By folk sector, Kleinman referred to non-professional specialists using a mixture of components spread throughout the entire medical field, although most of them are related to the popular sector. The folk sector can be divided into sacred and secular parts, although they often overlap.

Kleinman's tripartition offers insights into possible hierarchical classification; however, what Kleinman's and Leslie's concepts have in common is that they both relied on the idea of fixed health systems with a core. Additionally, Allopathy exists in almost all so-called non-Western countries and as such is always used as the point of reference for "the other" systems. This has produced a clear dichotomy between East and West and has obscured the fact that there is a strong tradition in European countries of heterogeneous practices encompassing lay healing, sorcery, witchcraft, and religious healing, among others.

In line with more recent anthropological work conducted by Sujatha (2007) and Sujatha and Abraham (2012), I neither conceptualize medical systems as delineated, definable and static over time, nor do I position health systems not closely related to Allopathy as "the other." Sujatha (ibid) dissolved fixed concepts about "scientific" traditions in the West and "folk healing" traditions in the East, since the Indian reality of medical knowledge is far more complex. Using Ayurveda and Siddha as examples, she claims that there are multiple layers of genres even within systems of knowledge. Through fieldwork in Tamil Nadu, Sujatha determined that medical lore, comprising basic concepts of health, body and disease, is not only held by medical practitioners (i.e., ayurvedic or Siddha doctors), but can also be found among laypeople. Sujatha calls this concept structural pluralism, which I will draw upon in the following chapters.

I define medical systems such as Naturopathy as cultural and cross-cultural systems of knowledge with underlying conceptions of personhood and self in relation to others, as well as specific definitions of health, disease and states in between. Medical systems are always evolving, in-process and multilayered. Therefore, they cannot be free of contradiction and gaps. Medical systems have multiple and heterogeneous epistemologies, and it is through this complex lens that social and medical reality is constructed.

3   Professional Alternatives: Institutionalized Non-Naturopathic
      Health Care in India

Health care in India is complex, influenced by colonial and post-colonial politics on the one hand and diverse lines of medical tradition on the other. The
range of options is also unique. For example, the Indian government's Ministry
of AYUSH, which was established to support multiple non-allopathic medical
systems, includes Ayurveda, Yoga, Naturopathy, Unani, Siddha, Homeopathy,
and Tibetan Medicine. Ayurveda, Unani and Siddha are often referred to as
"indigenous systems of medicine," while others, such as Homeopathy and
Naturopathy, are linked to European civilization and are thus perceived as
imported (Sujatha and Abraham 2009, Sujatha and Abraham 2012, Weiss 2009:
6). These systems co-exist in Indian society along with religious healing, folk
traditions, and of course Allopathy. The acceptance, appropriation, and contestation of several medical traditions over the course of centuries and their
hybridization with local variants highlight the flexibility of Indian systems
(Sujatha and Abrahams 2012). In the section below, I provide an overview on
the AYUSH systems of medicine.[1]

Ayurveda
Ayurveda has gained in popularity over the course of a few decades in both lay
and scholarly circles; indeed, one could fill libraries solely with the amount of
literature on Ayurveda that is produced by anthropologists alone. Ayurveda
has undergone many changes in recent decades, from what was once a set of
heterogeneous practices, loosely categorized under the term Ayurveda, to an
institutionalized health care system with scientific research methods and
standardized training (Langford 2002, Leslie 1976, Dunn 1976). Since there is no
exact foundation of Ayurveda but rather a number of historical interpretations, it is challenging to describe. In the following, I offer a short summary of
what is assigned, taught and understood today as "ayurvedic concepts," drawing from Wujastyk and Smith (2008) and Halliburton (2009, 2000).
    Ayurveda is based on classical texts such as the *Susrutha Samhita* and the
Caraka Samhita that were composed between 200 BC and 200 AD. The explanation of health and disease in Ayurveda is founded on a humoral theory of
constitutional balance and imbalance among various elements in the bodily
system. Human beings and every other aspect of the universe are comprised of
the *panchabuthas*, the five elements of earth, air, water, fire and ether. These
elements combine to form seven tissues (*dhatus*): chyle, blood, flesh, fat,
bone, marrow and semen. These tissues are further nourished by food. The

---

1   The infrastructure of the respective systems can be found in the appendix.

panchabuthas also combine to form the three *dosas*, called wind, fire and rain (*phlegm*) or *vata, pitta* and *kapha*. The *dosa* constitution of a person is given by birth and is known as *prakrti*, which literally means "natural or original form." These three humors exhibit some similarities with the ancient Greek teachings of Hippocrates. Zimmermann (1995) suggests that *dosa* can be conceptualized as a mnemonic device, as a way of thinking about the body. However, as Halliburton (2009) remarks, Sanskrit terms that are used in Ayurveda cannot easily be translated into other languages and therefore have no exact equivalent in English.

Diagnosis is provided by various methods depending on healer and context. Nowadays, common techniques include the inspection of urine, excrement, tongue and eyes, measurement of the pulse, and use of a stethoscope (Tirodkar 2008). A very common treatment is the *panchakarma*, a series of therapies with the aim of freeing the body from bad bodily fluids. Massages, enemas, therapeutic vomiting, nose showers and arteriotomies are common methods of cleansing the body (Svoboda 1995).

Legal recognition at the state level and the pursuit of greater integration into the existing medical establishment are reflected by the self-validation of ayurvedic medicine in publications and the professional medical fraternity. Although Ayurveda is known as an old tradition, Kaiser (1992) argues that it does not need to shy away from comparison with modern sciences such as Allopathy. On the contrary, Ayurveda seeks to combine an ancient Indian history with the modernity of lab technologies and doctors in white overalls. Anthropologists call this process the revivalism and modernization of Ayurveda (Brass 1972).

Although student associations undertake political activities to ensure that only college-educated and registered ayurvedic doctors are able to practice, traditional *vaidyas* (meaning non-college-trained practitioners) do still exist and practice despite their lack of visibility. Ayurveda's flexible system has made it possible to incorporate globalized concepts of disease and to adapt research methods that are normally found only within allopathic research. This is how Ayurveda has attempted to meet the expectations of modern patients who are used to allopathic diagnostic and technical equipment (Lang and Jansen 2010). The ayurvedic drug industry in particular is very successful in promoting and selling a huge variety of ayurvedic pharmaceuticals. There is an enormous market for these drugs because they are associated with promises of being more natural, "Indian" in their origins, and with fewer side effects than their allopathic versions. Thus, Ayurveda is booming with the hope for a holistic, smooth and pleasant way of healing (Banerjee 2004, Banerjee et al 2013, Ecks 2013, Halliburton 2003, Bode 2006).

This promise of a holistic approach is exactly what attracts medical tourists from both India and abroad. Kerala in particular is known for its ayurvedic resorts, which have become wellness temples offering pleasant ayurvedic treatments. Patients take the opportunity to combine this treatment with all manner of holidays. Medical tourism and its appropriation of ayurvedic concepts has been discussed elsewhere (Cyranski forthcoming, Cherukara & Manalel 2008). According to Spitzer (2009), for Indian tourists, the use of ayurvedic treatments for their ailments constitutes a specific expression of local identity. They adopt and use Ayurveda as a political project that *"entails the embodiment of political values"* (ibid: 141, citing Nichter 1996: 212).

Yoga

Yoga is central to the intellectual history of South Asia and, at the same time, it is an institutionalized medical system supported by AYUSH with its own colleges and opportunities to complete a PhD. In *Yoga in Modern India*, the anthropologist Joseph Alter (2004) examines the transmutation of Yoga from a philosophy to physical education, public health and institutionalized practice. He defines Yoga as follows:

> In essence Yoga holds that the world, as it is commonly perceived by the mind through self-consciousness, is an illusion based on ignorance. [...] The practice of Yoga is designed to transform illusion into reality by transcending ignorance and training the embodied mind to experience Truth (ibid:4).

Yoga shares some common ground with the *Samkhya* philosophy, although, as Alter points out, it has a different methodology and involvement of the body. In the context of medical pluralism in South India, Yoga holds a special position. Officially, it is attached to Naturopathy. It is therefore taught at naturopathic colleges and used in naturopathic hospitals, almost as an integral part of naturopathic theory. According to employees of AYUSH, Naturopathy and Yoga have been combined into one system because of their strongly-related ideologies and the fact that neither use medication in the classical sense. In addition, both rely on the *panchabutha* elementariness and pursue a state of detoxification and purgation. Although Yoga is attached to Naturopathy, its philosophical background also clearly resembles Siddha and Ayurveda. Yoga is taught to a certain degree in most Siddha colleges, while ayurvedic colleges normally have a separate Yoga department. It is also commonly used in the ayurvedic treatment of patients, be it in a hospital or at a health camp. It appears that Yoga is nowadays an integral part of all systems of medicine having any connection with *Samkhya* philosophy. The enormous success of Yoga in India and abroad over the last several decades as both a philosophy and physical fitness method has made it a powerful marker of Indian culture, identity and history.[2]

Unani & Siddha

Unani and Ayurveda have strongly influenced each other. Unani is also based on a humoral theory, but in contrast to Ayurveda, the doctrine holds that there are four different fluids in the body: phlegm, blood, yellow bile and black bile. These humors are generated during the process of digestion through the stomach. As in ayurvedic philosophy, health is only assured when these humors are balanced (Wujastyk 2003, Liebeskind 1995, Quaiser 2012a, 2012b). Unani medicine arrived in India with the introduction of Islam and forms the third largest medical system in contemporary India after Allopathy and Ayurveda.

Siddha, a medical system that evolved out of Tamil and Telugu texts in the south of India, is, according to Wujastyk (2003), "*primarily an esoteric, alchemical, and magical system, apparently strongly influenced by tantric thought and Ayurveda* [...]" (ibid: 31). Although anthropologists have written little about Siddha, it is the second most popular medical system in contemporary Tamil Nadu South India. The language of expression and history differs from Ayurveda, but the conceptual framework of Siddha is quite similar: the theory of *panchabutha* and *tridoshas* form the basic edifice (Wujastyk 2003, Weiss 2009). However, the concept of *chakras*, seven vital centers of energy, is more popular in Siddha than in Ayurveda. Five of these spots are associated with the *panchabutha*. Diagnostic methods are diverse: in addition to pulse diagnosis, a patient's urine, eyes, tongue and excrement are examined. Additionally, there is a methodological questioning of the patient. In Siddha medicine, the use of metal, especially mercury, and a substance called *muppu* is central to the treatment. The latter is seen to have the power to effect physical and spiritual transformation, heal disease and bestow immortality. Siddha holds a special

---

2   Only recently has a new discussion arisen concerning the commercialization and intellectual property of Yoga: In the beginning of the 21st century, Bikram Choudhury, one of the pioneers in commercializing Yoga in the U.S. and increasingly in Europe, sparked a huge controversy by claiming and aggressively enforcing broad copyrights for his sequences and style of Yoga *asanas*, or postures. As a consequence, in India hundreds of historians attested to the postures' historical authenticity and created a catalogue with the "original" postures in order to have a point of reference for future patent claims. However, Choudhury still insists on the copyright of his style of Yoga. Unfortunately, this discussion has not yet been dealt with in anthropology, although it provides a perfect example of the struggle for authenticity within Indian medical systems and traditions.

position in Indian society due to its strong connections to astrology and its alchemically-prepared medications (Alex 2010).

Both Unani and Siddha have been subject to the process of professionaliza-tion in recent decades (Siddha, e.g. Sujatha 2009, Unani, e.g. Leslie 1972). Additionally, both systems employ modern marketing strategies to sell their drugs (Weiss 2009, Liebeskind 1995, Bode 2006). Although their commercial-ization is not as permeating and visible as Ayurveda's aggressive drug marketing, Unani and Siddha medicines target their local consumers in their particular niches, with Unani more prevalent in the northern Indian regions and Siddha more common in the South.

Homeopathy

Homeopathy was invented in Germany by Samuel Hahnemann. Unlike most other medical systems, it is possible to fix the exact year Homeopathy emerged: 1796, the year when Hahnemann published his first article about an experi-ment he conducted on himself. The method of healing that this system follows is based on the simile-principle: this means that a disease can be healed with medication that evokes similar symptoms to the disease itself. Medications have a central role in Homeopathy: they are created through gradual attenua-tion of an active ingredient (*dilution*) before comminuting (*pulverization*) or agitation (*dynamization*). The latter process of agitation is necessary in order to let the material substance dissolve in the solution. The fundamental idea of Homeopathy is therefore contrary to allopathic medicine because it is theo-rized that the more diluted a substance is, the more potent it becomes. Ho-meopathy was brought to India by missionaries and began to spread throughout the country at the beginning of the 19th century (Frank 2004).

Tibetan Medicine

Tibetan Medicine (Sowa-Rigpa) was only incorporated into the AYUSH systems of medicine very recently. Demographic data collected in 2008 show that Tibetans constitute the largest refugee group in India. On account of this, it is no surprise that their medical practices, though not yet institutionalized, are now quite widespread and well-recognized. However, this is mainly the case in the North where Tibetans have settled, such as the well-known city of Dharamsala (Prost 2008). Since practitioners of Tibetan medicine have already become fairly professionalized in their field and their medications are adver-tised to the public, a strong move towards institutionalization is expected within the next few years.

4   The Institutionalization and Professionalization of the AYUSH
         Systems of Medicine

The Ministry of AYUSH officially dates back to 1969 when the *Department of Indian Systems of Medicine* (ISM) was founded. There was no separation between single medical systems; all were combined to a certain degree and supposedly protected by the ISM and therefore by the Ministry of Health & Family Welfare. It was not until 1978 that all of the so-called drugless systems were separated and guidelines were formulated. In 1995, Homeopathy was officially added and the name was changed to the *Department of Indian Systems of Medicine & Homeopathy* (ISM&H). The department represented all of the medical systems that were regarded either as indigenous or as now part of the Indian tradition: Ayurveda, Siddha, Unani, Homeopathy and therapies such as Naturopathy and Yoga. In 2003, it was renamed the *Department of Ayurveda, Yoga and Naturopathy, Unani, Siddha and Homeopathy* (AYUSH). The legal acceptance of Naturopathy by the government as a concrete medical system is considered to be a milestone. Amchi/Sowa-Rigpa (Tibetan Medicine) was included in 2010. In 2014, the department was recognized as an independent Ministry. Its objectives include improving educational standards and programs, strengthening so-called evidence-based research programs, promoting the cultivation of medicinal plants, and enhancing pharmacopoeial standards (AYUSH 2016a-d, Priya 2012). In practice, this is implemented through different Ministry bodies working to enhance research, education and awareness (i.e. national campaigns) for all of the medical systems. AYUSH funds hospitals, health camps, events, media work and colleges.

Several steps were necessary in order to render the institutionalization of non-allopathic medical systems possible: The planning phase through the *Medicine Central Council Act* in 1970, followed in 1973 by the inclusion of Homeopathy through the *Homeopathy Central Council Act*. The latter made it possible to delineate practitioners who underwent formal, standardized education from so-called quacks. The *Delhi Medical Council*, founded in 1998 immediately after the passage of the *Delhi Medical Council Act* in 1997, is the new platform through which doctors register. The primary intention of this registration system is to protect patients.[3]

---

3 According to the Medical Council Association, the punishment for malpractice or quackery is one year of imprisonment and/or a fine of one thousand rupees. The Association estimates that there are still approximately 30,000 quacks in India, including the ones that work in allopathic institutions as nurses, dental hygienists and even doctors.

Nowadays, all AYUSH systems except Sowa-Rigpa have AYUSH-supported colleges as well as independent colleges.[4] Each system is subject to a standardized syllabus with a unitary degree: Bachelor of Ayurvedic Medicine and Surgery (BAMS), Bachelor of Siddha Medicine and Surgery (BSMS), Bachelor of Unani Medicine and Surgery (BUMS), Bachelor of Naturopathy and Yogic Sciences (BNYS), and Bachelor of Homeopathic Medicines and Surgery (BHMS). The courses last between 4.5 and 5.5 years, which corresponds to the Indian allopathic Bachelor of Medicine and Bachelor of Surgery (MBBS). Most AYUSH courses integrate foundational allopathic knowledge such as first aid, anatomy, chemistry or biology as basic studies of the human body alongside their field-specific education. As the title of their respective degrees show, Ayurveda, Siddha, Unani and Homeopathy students even learn surgery to a certain degree. The courses are formally brought into line with the allopathic MBBS by establishing undergraduate training and postgraduate training. To qualify for the university courses one must have completed at least twelve years of schooling in science subjects and have passed the *All India Pre-Medical Test*, consisting of 25% chemistry, 25% physics and 50% biology questions.

The institutions of the Indian state are striving to formalize and standardize all medical practices. Several reasons may underlie the motivation to legitimize Indian medical systems such as Ayurveda and Unani: first, legitimization reassures patients that they are in trusted hands; second, it proves to other medical systems that their respective approaches are scientific and therefore reasonable; and lastly and perhaps most importantly, it demonstrates their professional standards to doctors and patients abroad. Health tourism is an important factor: Since it has become a significant source of business in India (Cheruka and Manalel 2008), conveying a professional image externally is absolutely necessary.

5   The Embodiment of Naturopathic Experience: Some Notes on Methodology

I began my research with an interest in the ways that "depression" is hybridized with local concepts and idioms of mental distress in South India. Along with my colleague at the time, Claudia Lang, I conducted fieldwork in various medical institutions in Kerala, such as Ayurveda psychiatric hospitals and colleges, psychological health centers, Hindu temples, charismatic retreat centers and

---

4   The following summary of education and registration of Indian practitioners is taken from the website of the Central Council for Indian Medicine (CCIM 2014).

Muslim places of healing. We were interested in how the creolization of psychiatric, psychological, physiological, social and cosmological idioms of distress fashion patients' embodied idioms of distress.

During that period I became acquainted with Indian Naturopathy through our first translator. I was already a regular guest in homes of naturopathic practitioners, and had listened to their opinions about depression, health and disease. Naturopathic theories and practices seemed both familiar and alien to me. The familiarity originated from my childhood experiences in Bavaria where my father underwent Kneipp's water treatments and followed his ideas of a balanced diet. At the same time, the strangeness resulted from a divergent systematization of naturopathic theory that became immediately apparent to me.

My fieldwork was staggered in three phases. My aim was to paint a picture of the heterogeneity of naturopathic practices and theories by means of a multi-sited ethnography, following the conflict between two divergent naturopathic ideologies (Marcus 1995). First, I undertook an exploratory segment from July through September 2009, where I established initial contacts, conducted first interviews and performed background research on the ways in which Naturopathy is presented in newspapers and books published by Naturopaths. In the second phase, from December 2009 through March 2010, I spent most of my time in hospitals: First in the Gandhiji Naturopathy Hospital (GNH) in Thrissur, then in the Nature Life Hospital (NLH) in Kozhikode, and finally, in the Mahatma Gandhi Nature Cure Center (MNCC) in Bakkalam. I spent approximately one month at each during that time. However, during these stays, I heard quite a bit from practitioners and patients about Universal Good Life Ashram (UGLA) in Sivasailam, so I decided to extend my research for an additional three weeks in the third phase of research, from December 2010 through March 2011. The remainder of my time was allocated to conducting background research to clarify the context of Naturopathy in South India. Specifically, I visited all relevant institutions such as the National Institute of Naturopathy (NIN) in Pune, the Yoga University SVASYA near Bangalore, the psychiatric hospital NIMHANS in Bangalore, the AYUSH offices, the Central Council for Research in Yoga and Naturopathy (CCRYN), and the All India Nature Cure Federation (AINCF) in Delhi, as well as the Indian Systems of Medicine (ISM) offices in Thiruvananthapuram. Moreover, I conducted a number of interviews and learned naturopathic techniques in the SDM College of Naturopathy and Yogic Science near Mangalore and the JSS College of Naturopathy and Yogic Science in Coimbatore. In addition to the four hospitals in which I conducted my research, I visited more than fifteen other naturopathic hospitals and ashrams as well as nature-cure camps in South India and Delhi (Map 1).

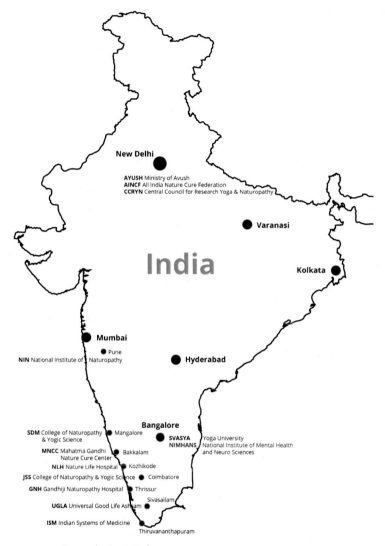

New Delhi

AYUSH Ministry of Avush
AINCF All India Nature Cure Federation
CCRYN Central Council for Research Yoga & Naturopathy

Varanasi

India   Kolkata

Mumbai

● Pune
NIN National Institute of Naturopathy   Hyderabad

Bangalore

SDM College of Naturopathy ● Mangalore   ● **SVASYA** Yoga University
& Yogic Science   **NIMHANS** National Institute of Mental Health
MNCC Mahatma Gandhi ● Bakkalam   and Neuro Sciences
Nature Cure Center
NLH Nature Life Hospital ● Kozhikode
JSS College of Naturopathy & Yogic Science ● Coimbatore
GNH Gandhiji Naturopathy Hospital ● Thrissur
Sivasailam
UGLA Universal Good Life Ashram ●

ISM Indian Systems of Medicine
Thiruvananthapuram

MAP 1   *Research sites in India*

Hospital fieldwork is quite a paradoxical mission. There is the methodological challenge of being a participant observer, which in a hospital setting means
being either the patient, the doctor, the bystander, the nurse or the treatment
assistant (Wind 2008). All of these positions have their problems: Being a
patient can be an impossible task, since most of the time the ethnographers
are not sick. Researchers have posed as patients in the past,[5] but this raises

5   For example in the famous cases of Rosenhan (1973) and Caudill (1958) in psychiatric hospi-

clear ethical questions. Playing the role of a doctor also poses difficulties since most of us do not have two courses of education, with some enviable exceptions such as Zaman (2005), who was an allopathic doctor from Bangladesh conducting research in a Bangladeshi hospital. Similarly, to be an assistant also requires specific expertise. My ideal role would have been that of bystander, but unfortunately (or fortunately) none of my friends ever got sick enough or decided to seek treatment in a naturopathic hospital. I was not able to join the staff, the doctors, the patients, the bystanders or the visitors at the same time and still have an overall picture as is expected in an ethnography.

I tried to resolve this dilemma by assuming different positions at different points in time: In the first hospital in Thrissur, the GNH, I was given the status of a medical intern, who was allowed to bring in food from outside and experience a doctor's perspective. This was only possible because the hospital is a teaching hospital and they receive interns regularly. However, my research efforts were restricted due to my lack of knowledge on Naturopathy and Malayalam and the general outsider position I always held. This was the only place where I was not allowed to take a look in the medical files or make audio recordings; I was told that the machine was not very "natural" and could be harmful.

At all of the other research sites, I underwent every treatment advised by my naturopathic doctors. Nature Life Hospitals are organized in a comparatively egalitarian way, which makes it easy to gather information. Most people there, whether employees, doctors or patients, prompt each other to share. Additionally, the hospital is accustomed to healthy visitors, such as friends meeting for conferences, travelers, or ordinary people who want a break from their (mostly urban) life. Altogether I fasted on water and coconut juice for about fifteen days. I lived on raw fruits and vegetables for weeks. I sweated in steam baths and got rolled in banana leaves on the roof of a house, I received more-or-less pleasant massages, I was wrapped in wet clothes and mud packs. Since it was said to be useful, I received a daily skin rub consisting of a mixture of turmeric and other herbs. Part of the treatment was a two-hour Yoga course every morning at five o'clock, which I joined. My diagnoses switched between lifestyle-improvement and a minor skin disease called urticaria, from which I had suffered for over five years. Sometimes I felt horrible and hungry, being wet, sweaty, and yellow-skinned from the turmeric paste.

---

tals, or more recently by van der Geest and Sarkodie (1999) in a Ghanaian hospital and Scheper-Hughes (2004) in the case of U.S. organ transplants.

All in all, studying Naturopathy did not always turn out to be very pleasant. During my field research in the hospitals I had to adapt myself to whatever "living a natural life" meant in that specific place. Taking part in all of these procedures as a patient, while still retaining the possibility of joining doctors for the rounds and looking at case reports, gave me closer insight to practitioners and provided me with an embodied understanding of what patients experience.

Although I studied Malayalam for quite a while, when it came to the life history details of monolingual Malayalam-speaking patients, it was necessary to work with translators. Many patients traveled for their treatment from Tamil Nadu, Maharashtra or even Punjab, which increased the language difficulties enormously. However, the practitioners without exception were well-aware of English rhetoric and so were most of the patients.

The research generated an enormous amount of data and materials, including journals, magazines, articles, videotapes, and transcriptions of over one hundred interviews. Most of the interviews were semi-structured, but there were also narrative interviews with practitioners, patients, relatives, theorists and political activists. Sometimes the demarcations between the latter two could not clearly be identified. My interactions with informants have not been constrained by time or place; through modern media such as the Internet, Facebook and email, as well as telephone calls and even letters, I am still in contact with many people in the field of Naturopathy in India, tracing their stories and watching their development.

6   Outline of Chapters

This book is divided into two main sections. The first two chapters, including this one, outline the genesis and development of Naturopathy in South India in order to provide a basic understanding of its current position and role. The second section comprises a social science analysis of the configurations of contemporary South Indian Naturopathy. While Chapters One and Two primarily make use of historical sources, the analysis in Chapters Three through Seven are based upon recently-collected ethnographic material.

Chapter Two, *The Embodiment of Resistance: (Dis)continuities in Indian Naturopathy*, explores the eclectic position of South Indian Naturopathy in the historical context of worldwide flows. I link its development to the politico-medical situation during colonialism, as basic principles of South Indian Naturopathy were defined as a response or frequently as acts of resistance.

Practitioners at the time drew upon the teachings of German naturopathic pioneers to develop an alternative to the biopower of Allopathy. Medical treatment thereby became part of the political battlefield, with the body employed as the main weapon in this struggle.

Chapter Three, *Evidence versus Experience: Two Streams of Naturopathy in South India*, examines the separation of the naturopathic movement into two competing branches in contemporary South India. Professionally-trained Naturopaths strive for what I term "scientification," emphasizing academic research and education. Their ambition is to institutionalize Naturopathy as a standardized, evidence-based system of medicine. On the other hand, psycho-nutritionals consider experience to be the most important source of knowledge. They uphold the banner of resistance against globalization and espouse a coherent ideology of simplicity, transparency and empowerment. Both groups significantly draw upon German and Indian naturopathic legacy, but hold very different interpretations.

Until this point I have examined naturopathic theory separate from its implementation and daily practices. However, in Chapter Four, *Naturopathic Spaces: On Nutrition, Substances and Psychological Integration*, ethnographic data carry us directly into the wards and dining rooms of naturopathic hospitals. The daily routines of two separate hospitals, one professional and the other psycho-nutritional, illuminate the different meanings and emphases attached to the treatments. I categorize these treatments into three modalities: nutritional therapy, substance-bases applications, and psychological integration. This chapter compares the differing priorities accorded to these modalities and, based upon the concept of the hospital as a naturopathic space, it explores the conclusions that one can draw from professional versus psycho-nutritional hospitals.

Chapter Five, *Naturopathic Actors: Between Ideology and Practice*, draws upon clinical staff biographies and observations to investigate if and how naturopathic ideology is reflected in their motivations, beliefs, and hierarchical organization. Two areas of friction are of particular relevance for both professional and psycho-nutritional staff: First, the border between hospital life and the private spheres of practitioners, and second, the implementation of an egalitarian ideology in the social organization of the hospital.

Chapter Six, *The Logic of Labeling: Diagnostics and Naturopathy*, describes the processes involved in the delineation of patients' diseases. It identifies the roles of diverse actors during the rather brief periods of hospital admission and daily rounds. In both contexts, practitioners and patients use allopathic knowledge and language to categorize the reasons for the latter's stay. The shifting relevance of diagnostic knowledge in Naturopathy has a critical impact on some patients' social lives outside the hospital – for instance, those with stigmatizing diseases such as mental illness.

The social context of patients' everyday lives is also at the heart of the last chapter of this book, *The Efforts of Freedom: Patients' Role in Achieving Medical Independence*. This chapter investigates the reasons for patients' frequent hospital readmissions as they strive for treatment success, despite Naturopathy's ideological promise of empowerment and independence. I analyze the medical narratives of several patient cases to learn more about the actual transferability of naturopathic treatments to their homes following their hospital stay. I learn that being free of symptoms – and perhaps disease – does not break their tie to the naturopathic hospital.

The Embodiment of Resistance: (Dis)continuities in Indian Naturopathy

The former schoolteacher Ramakrishnan was both a well-known and enigmatic figure in South India; several rumors circulated around his life and death. During my initial field research in Kerala in naturopathic hospitals, both practitioners and patients repeatedly referred to Ramakrishnan and his approach to health and disease when I asked how they began to learn about Naturopathy. Interviewees often equated his influence on the practice of Naturopathy to that of Gandhi. He drew enough interest so that people both with and without disease, who were interested in non-invasive healing methods or in nationalistic movements, visited him in his ashram, Sivasailam Ashram,[1] during his lifetime or traveled there after his death.

Sivasailam Ashram is now considered to be the first naturopathic hospital in South India. It took me quite a while to track down the exact location of his activities, since it has changed considerably: it is now a 30-bed hospital run by one BNYS doctor, the son of Ramakrishnan, and it employs two PGs. Serious diseases such as ulcers, cancer, diabetes and heart problems are treated in addition to obesity and migraines. Rooms are allotted to the patient either for 500 rupees a day inclusive of food and treatments, or for an additional cost with air conditioning. The surrounding property is green and picturesque, with cows, cats and dogs roaming freely, very unlike other naturopathic hospitals, and very unlike most of the hospitals I have seen in India. Banana and coconut trees dominate the visible flora, and there is a small pond with a small stream on the side. There are several mismatched buildings on the property, obviously built in different decades: small run-down huts, modern-looking two-story buildings with fresh paint, and a new building for treatments. An arena in the middle of the ashram hints at the events that have been held there in the past, such as speeches. On the side there is a Yoga hall with four modern gym machines and a number of mats, ready to be used for *asanas*. However, despite the modernity, patients, visitors and employees still refer to Ramakrishnan as their motivation for staying in the ashram. On the main building, there is a sign in Tamil quoting him (Figure 1):

---

1   For more information on the ashram as it is today, see Internet source UGLA 2016.

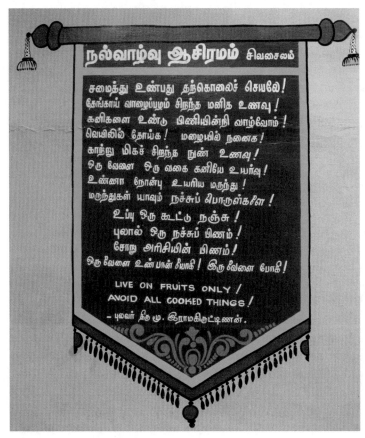

FIGURE 1   *Sign in Tamil – UGLA*

Cooked food is like a suicide attempt
Coconut and banana are the best food humans can have
Let us eat fruits and live without any disease
Feel the sunlight
Drench in the rain
Air is the best food
Any time of day fruit is better
Fasting is one of the best medicines
All English medicines are toxic substances
Salt is part of the poison
Meat is a toxic corpse
Rice is the dead body of the paddy
Eat healthy food twice a day.

Ramakrishnan was probably born in 1931 or 1932 and has become the mythical hero of Naturopathy throughout Kerala, Tamil Nadu and Maharashtra. Ramakrishnan discovered Naturopathy through Tamil writings on nature cures and Gandhi's influence, and soon modified his lifestyle into what he referred to as a "natural way." Ramakrishnan wanted to counter the emerging consumption of post-colonial products and values and exemplify a "local life." He became famous in South India for his experiments with fruits and his promotion of health and naturalism. He conducted several health camps and other activities and invited like-minded people from all over India to attend. Apparently some people even stayed for years. For the purpose of detoxification, every cohabitant had to go on a three-day water fast after his or her arrival. In the 1970s, Ramakrishnan bought land with the help of donations and opened the current ashram. In the early days, Ramakrishnan, the patients and visitors slept in the open air and took their baths in the forest, a story still recounted euphorically today by people in the ashram. He taught school every morning to financially support his activities but spent the rest of the day at the ashram.

From the 1970s onwards, Ramakrishnan tried several variations of diet: First, he and his followers consumed ten bananas and one coconut, the most common fruits of the area, over the course of the day. Mr. Chandra, a follower of Ramakrishnan who came as a patient in 1974 and is now on the staff, explains the logic behind the choice of bananas and coconuts:

> Ramakrishnan divided the food system into five varieties. The food that is cultivated below the ground like potato and carrots is meant for pigs and other things because they can dig it and take the food and the leaves can be eaten by cattle. That is also not good for man. Vegetables are for insects like for worms and grains and pulses and nuts are meant for the birds. Milk is only for the baby cow. For man there is only coconut and banana.

Cohabitants of the ashram planted trees and cultivated different kinds of fruits. Later, Ramakrishnan integrated other elements into the diet, such as dates, juices and mixed vegetables. As I was told by his son and Mr. Chandra, at one point Ramakrishnan consumed only one date for 10 or 15 days. Since he could still handle his daily routine, he cut down to half a coconut for a period of four or five years. Afterwards he dieted completely, which is referred to as "dry fasting." It is said in the ashram that Ramakrishnan did not drink water for 38 days straight. After that he consumed a small amount of juice. He could not digest it and died from the effects of diarrhea on March 26th, 1990. Mr. Chandra refers to Ramakrishnan's ambition as "*scientific instinct,*" because "*he wanted to do research on nature, food and health and demonstrate that there is no need for the consumption of too many things."* Mr. Chandra is convinced that within three or four generations of minimizing food, people would be able to live on only air without any consequences to their health; Ramakrishnan had already taken the first steps in this direction but made the mistake of going back to consumption. His life and death have remained a source of interest and discussion to this day for patients staying in his hospital, as well as for staff and practitioners in South India. Many of my informants pointed to his inspirational attitude and spoke of him as a mythical figure. Universal Good Life Ashram (UGLA) is still a popular place for naturopathic treatment particularly because many patients are still familiar with Ramakrishnan and visit the ashram regularly. Ramakrishnan devoted his life to his experiments, which were intended to prove the efficacy of Naturopathy. Although he did not publish works himself,[2] he strove to be a model and to attract followers. However, his approach to diet – a completely minimalistic intake of dates, bananas and coconut – is seen as too radical by most contemporary Naturopaths.

The second famous Naturopath I want to introduce here is C.R.R. Varma (1929-1999). Most of my informants are convinced that it was Varma who fostered a wide audience for Naturopathy in Kerala. He was an engineer who gave up his profession after encountering the Naturopath Swaminathan from New Delhi. Varma spent his life traveling through Kerala at regular intervals and gave lectures about health, disease and nature. He refused to build a treatment center but instead ran several clinics where people could receive counseling on their state of health and potential modifications to their lifestyle. The most famous center can be found close to Guruvayoor in North Kerala but there are still naturopathic centers running in several cities in his honor. Varma wrote six books in Malayalam that still serve as the educational base for Naturopaths in Kerala and South India. In these books, Varma claimed on the basis of Louis Kuhne that there is only one disease, the toxification of the body, but since *"ordinary people find this difficult to accept"* (Varma 2001b), he went on to detail how to approach common issues such as boils, acne, hemorrhage, dizziness, lack of appetite, itching, fatigue, mumps, tonsillitis, fever, loose stool, headaches, colds and vomiting. He explained that the main treatment methods are fasting and water therapy, two therapies that can relieve all discomfort. Although the relationship between the theory citing unity of disease and Varma's subsequent analysis of etiology, symptoms and healing methods for various ailments may seem to be contradictory, it is quite a common theme in

---

2 Ramakrishnan's younger brother, Dr. M. Aanaiappan, published two books on his legacy (Aanaiappan 1999, 2000). Ramakrishnan's son is also about to publish a book on his life and approach to Naturopathy.

the naturopathic approach, with its roots in the teachings of Kuhne (Kumar 2005).

In other books (Varma 2001a, 2001c), Varma expanded on his ideas about nutrition, integrated treatments with those derived from the Indian concept of the "five elements," and discussed the chemical composition of carbohydrates and the chemical reaction that takes place in combination with saliva. His books have a very ideological, insistent tone but are still concerned with nature-based scientific knowledge (Kumar 2005). Varma considered a change in lifestyle unavoidable in order to live according to naturopathic principles. He therefore recommended local and unprocessed food and the use of naturopathic treatment methods. He did not see himself as a doctor but rather as a mouthpiece of Gandhi's legacy. His main aim was to make Malayalis aware of their own responsibility in matters of health. Political motives were not explicitly communicated but can be inferred since he urged his fellow countrymen to live off of local products.

The anecdotes of these two famous figures of South Indian Naturopathy are neither rare nor unique in the history of the transmission of naturopathic knowledge from abroad to and throughout India. Naturopathy has become very popular in India nowadays, in stark contrast to other countries in Asia. An easy explanation for this phenomenon might be the general openness to pluralistic medical therapies in India. However, this argument falls short and does not consider the specific historical circumstances and turning points with regard to naturopathic theory and practice that coalesced to promote the development of Naturopathy in India as it is unique to a non-European country. The rest of this chapter traces the continuities, discontinuities, dissemination and integration of naturopathic theories and practices in India. All medical systems have developed particular conceptions of bodies, health and well-being; my aim in this chapter is to trace the latter through history. My starting point is the initial position of colonialism in India and its impact on health systems. The colonial biopower had a major influence on the nature of the independence and nationalist movement with Gandhi as its leading player. Because Gandhi and other first-generation Indian Naturopaths drew heavily from European Naturopaths to legitimize their resistance, the subsequent part explains the significance of this European alternative movement. The last part analyzes the conceptual synthesis that has become characteristic of the contemporary theory and practice of Indian Naturopathy – and therefore also important to the opus of C.R.R. Varma and Ramakrishnan.

1   The Biopolitics of Colonialism and Medicine in India

In order to understand the backdrop into which Naturopathy was introduced, it is necessary to provide a brief illustration of the relationship between colonialism and medicine in India. Writing history on colonialism is not an easy task since "*one must write against the logic of imperialism by refusing to let the trajectory of modern nationalism define the structure of history,*" as Alter (2005: 4-5) puts it. Therefore, an analysis can only be implemented by default from the perspective of the adoption of allopathic medicine. As in many other geographical contexts, there are few writings from the perspective of the colonized.[3] Medicine was not, of course, the only important example of the appropriation, contestation and negotiation of hierarchies in the process of colonization. However, due to specific local circumstances, it played a major role in the development of the constitution of power in India, and in fact became an embattled field between the British colonizers and the Indian locals. David Arnold (2000, 1993) emphasizes the impact of medicine on Western scientific thought and actions during colonialism, and argues that this impact was due to the English interest in investigating their new environment and the direct points of interaction with Indian cultural and social life. Indeed, the number of surgeons and other allopathic practitioners in India, as well as zoologists and geologists, was enormous during the colonial period and provided many areas of contact with the local population.

Mark Harrison (2001) provides a useful picture of the relationship between European and Indian medicine. He identifies five different stages in the encounters between colonialists and the Indian population. In its first stage, when the first Portuguese arrived prior to 1670, the relationship was on equal footing. Europeans were even eager to learn from the Indians and shared a similar view of the body "*as being composed of elements or humours (the exact number depending on the system), which displayed qualities of moisture, warmth, cold, dryness and so forth*" (ibid: 40). The idea of unbalanced humors as a source of disease was quite common in central Europe until well into the 1800s, drawing upon the ancient Greek paradigm (Wujastyk 2003, King 2013).

However, in the second stage of colonization between 1670 and 1770, that incipient respect disappeared due to a shift in the Western paradigm following new discoveries in anatomy and blood circulation. The disparity between European and Indian ideas on medicine began to grow: Europeans regarded

---

3   Attempts to view colonial processes from another perspective, from the perspective of the colonized, are exemplified by authors involved in Subaltern Studies: for example, Arnold (2000) or Prakash (1990).

their own medical system as scientific, based on rationality and observation, while they rejected Indian medicine as being traditional and therefore backward. An asymmetrical relationship developed in which Indian medicine was regarded as inferior. It was also during this period that the *Indian Medical Service* was founded. It served as the official allopathic organization and established provincial medical boards with two surgeons each throughout the country. These boards were primarily established to cater to the needs of English soldiers stationed in India (Arnold 2000).

In the period between 1770 and approximately 1820 – referred to by Harrison as the third phase – British scholars known as the "Orientalists" (in the sense defined by Edward Said) began to systematically translate and analyze Sanskrit texts. In a re-creation of India's history, the Orientalists postulated that India had a classical past and an enormous cultural knowledge, and that it was up to them to recover it in an attempt to avoid a cultural decline. This could only happen, they argued, if Indians were freed from their "superstitious beliefs" and became more "scientific." The Orientalists were opposed by "Anglicists," who were not interested in the study of Indian values and believed that for any societal progress to be made, a shift towards the British lifestyle was required.

For the analysis of contemporary and former Naturopathy in India, however, the fourth phase is the most important. After 1820 the contact between English and Indian practitioners intensified. The British were very fond of collecting and implementing knowledge from the Indian *vaidyas* and other medical practitioners, particularly in the field of medicinal plants. They strove to identify the "useful" elements of indigenous therapies and in their view these were limited mostly to drugs. At the same time, new discoveries and the elaboration of scientific methods taking place in Europe and the United States bolstered the confidence of Western scientists. These developments made their way slowly into the colonies of these imperial powers. Probably due to the rapid development of material Western medicine, such as pills and injections, the appropriation of Indian medical knowledge was essentially restricted to drugs. The British excluded therapeutic techniques and therefore did not integrate Western and Indian bodily concepts or notions.

The gradual fixation of colonial power in Indian institutions was fostered by the formation of hierarchies of medical knowledge: the colonialists established the first Ayurveda and Unani teaching institutions in vernacular languages with the requirement to teach at least a minimum of allopathic knowledge, which reflected its growing dominance. These teaching institutions were meant to supplement the limited number of English doctors, who also had administrative responsibilities and were constantly at risk of sickness. Apparently, courses in Ayurveda and Unani were offered more for practical

reasons than to persuade people of their effectiveness: they were intended to
attract and hopefully convince *vaidyas* and other kinds of medical practitioners of the superiority of allopathic medicine. Those interested were offered
further training and employment within the institutions of the colonial regime.
Arnold summarizes the relationship between Allopathy and Indian medicine
in that period as follows:

> Western medicine after 1835 was taken as the hallmark of a higher civili-
> zation, a sign of the moral purpose and legitimacy of colonial rule in
> India, just as indigenous medical ideas and practices could be casually
> equated with ignorance and barbarism (Arnold 1993: 57).

The primary focus of medical education was therefore on allopathic practices.
By the end of the 19th century, quite a number of Indian doctors had graduated
from courses in allopathic medicine. During this phase, the political issue of
vaccination arose, a contentious debate and one to which contemporary
Naturopaths still refer. For them the imposition of vaccination, even in the
present time, is equal to the absolute escalation of biogovernmentality as mas-
sive bodily control by the government.

   With the practice of vaccination, colonialists dismissed folk practices rather
than the techniques of Ayurveda and Unani. At the time, a common method of
protecting against smallpox was variolation, the intended exposure to smallpox contagion with the intention of immunization. Apparently this practice
occasionally led to serious cases of smallpox that threatened to turn into epi-
demics. The British founded the *Smallpox Commission* in order to suppress
what was, in their view, the very cruel and murderous practice of variolation
and accordingly to promote a shift to vaccination. Their actions were given
legal justification with the passage of vaccination legislation in the 1870-80s,
through which variolation simply became illegal. However, a problem arose:
the vaccination serum was not available in India and had to be imported. Thus,
these laws were rather difficult to implement. Although English medical advis-
ers disagreed about whether it would be preferable to bring variolation under
state control, the colonialists' mistrust of the local handling of the practice
preponderated. The acceptance of vaccination, on the other hand, did not
meet with resounding success within the Indian population. Disregarding the
religious significance variolation seemed to possess for Indians, the anti-vacci-
nation sentiments were fueled in part by the simple dislike of the "colonial
mark" that vaccinations left on their skin and the perception that it was
*"ungodly and offensively polluting in its crude transmission of body fluids from
one individual to another"* (Arnold 2000: 74). Brimnes (2004) argues that the

practice of variolation was not a common method in the South of India. Instead, people in that region, especially high-caste Brahmins, resisted all kinds of immunization, whether it was variolation or vaccination, since both were suspicious to them.[4]

Although Harrison identified the period after 1880 as the last phase, otherwise known as the *Rediscovery of Indian Medicine*, he remains uncertain about whether or not the colonialists' interest in Indian medicine is reflective of *"nothing more than the appropriation of indigenous knowledge for the purpose of demand"* (Harrison 2001: 38). Nevertheless, what is certain at this point is that the British colonizers systematically oppressed indigenous medical practices for the purpose of ensuring colonial domination. The expression of this colonial power is not only political, institutional and administrative, but is profoundly bodily in its facilitation of certain medical techniques, drugs and concepts and the abolishment of others. In 1993, Arnold published his book entitled *Colonization of the Body*, which corroborates the immense corporality of colonialism. He described the basic principles of colonizing the body as follows:

> First there is the nature of colonialism itself. Colonial rule built up an enormous battery of texts and discursive practices that concerned themselves with the physical being of the colonized (and, no less critically though the interconnection is too seldom recognized, of the colonizers implanted in their midst). Colonialism used – or attempted to use – the body as a site for the construction of its own authority, legitimacy, and control (ibid: 8).

---

4   While smallpox was familiar to the British due to its occurrence in Europe, the containment of other "tropical" diseases such as malaria posed more of a challenge, especially for research purposes. Efforts were made, though, to link malaria with specific topographic and environmental factors such as the climate and the monsoon. A similar mystery was the occasional outbreak of cholera, which became an increasing danger for both the Indian and the British population. British researchers assumed meteorological as well as cultural and social factors (e.g. religious festivals or famine) as reasons for the epidemic prevalence of cholera. Even the identification of the bacillus in a water tank by Robert Koch in 1884 did not convince the colonialists, so entrenched was their belief in environmental factors (Arnold 2000). The issue of smallpox differs from the more "mysterious and tropical" diseases, including "fevers" such as malaria or "fluxes" such as cholera, with regard to its occurrence (India and Europe) and the colonial idea of its easy prevention. For this reason malaria and cholera were less politicized than the vaccination against smallpox. In this matter, the British wanted to show the clear superiority of their medicine and beyond (Brimnes 2004).

In Arnold's argument, the local response to this attempt to dominate the Indian body is manifested in the discourse of disease and healing in colonial India and, of course, in the resistance to vaccination and adherence to local practices such as variolation. Arnold drew upon the logic of Foucault when he described the political repression through the means of medical control by the rulers. Indeed, the institutionalization of Ayurveda, Unani and allopathic practices contributed to the disciplining power of the colonial state. The collision of British and preexisting heterogeneous healing methods can be defined as "epistemic violence" (Mukharji 2011), and refers to the essentially asymmetric blending and synchronistic delineation of certain elements of the various medical epistemologies – also creating new possibilities, logics and modalities of the body and healing by overhauling others (see also Kumar 1997).

2   Disseminating Naturopathic Knowledge in India

Gandhi was one of the actors creating new paradigms and implementing them as a logical consequence to the imperialism of the body. Unfortunately, Arnold underestimated the role of Gandhi in generating local resistance to colonial medicine, claiming that "*Gandhi's critique was as rare as it was radical*" (ibid: 187). Yet, Gandhi's total disavowal of Western imperialism was intended precisely to free the body from colonization; his ideas have a long history and are gaining even greater influence today. His young adult years were marked by emigration to England and South Africa. Therefore he was originally not part of any Indian-based anti-colonialism movement (Alter 2000) and he observed from a distance the gradual rise in Allopathy's influence in India.

There is plenty of literature on the life and legacy of Gandhi, most of it dealing with political issues, social relationships and, of course, his use of non-cooperation and non-violence as methods of resistance to imperial power.[5] This section, however, will primarily focus on Gandhi's ideas about diet, his adoption of Naturopathy following encounters with other medical systems and the connection of health and body with the political sphere in building

---

5   For example, see Som (2004) for a discussion of the political relationships between Gandhi, Bose and Nehru. Historical approaches can be found in Nanda (2002), Das (2005) or Scalmer (2011). Erikson (1969) provided a psychoanalytical study of Gandhi's motives and the notion of Truth. Erikson focused on a 1918 dispute between mill owners and workers and includes Gandhi's autobiographical notes as well as testimonies of contemporary witnesses. Kakar (1990) published a study about Gandhi's sexual and non-sexual relationships with women, also using a psychoanalytical approach.

the nation. I refer to Gandhi's approach to the latter trio as the *embodiment of resistance*, since Gandhi's struggle for Truth, home rule (*swaraj*), and his effort to maintain his own health as well as the health of the nation was strongly inscribed in his body. I regard Gandhi as the main collector and most heard medium of naturopathic flows, drawing on Appadurai (2002, 1996, see Chapter One).

Diet

In his autobiography, Gandhi described the stages that led him from being a vegetarian in India to engaging in radical fasting periods for political ends.[6] Although Gandhi experimented with meat-eating in his childhood, he grew up in a primarily vegetarian household in Gujarat. While studying law in England, he joined the English Vegetarian Society to meet like-minded people. Gandhi was a strong advocate of a so-called simple life. His idealistic attempts to lead life by minimalistic means started in South Africa, where, in tribute to the famous writer, he founded Tolstoy Farm, a place for people of all religions practicing subsistence farming. There Gandhi strove to live like a *brahmachari*, the realization of the *brahman*, a way of life that includes a special diet, occasional fasting, celibacy and exercise. He experimented with diet and finally decided that "*the brahmachari's food should be limited, simple, spiceless, and, if possible, uncooked*" (Gandhi 2013 [1927]: 193). Gandhi also attempted to control thoughts, lusts, words and deeds. The goal of his experiment was self-restraint with regard to food and sexual activities, and the attainment of complete self-control.[7]

Naturopathy and Other Medical Systems

Gandhi's first application of naturopathic treatment also took place on this farm when his son had an attack of typhoid combined with pneumonia. Although the doctor strongly recommended eggs and chicken, Gandhi refused this treatment and instead gave his son hip baths and other hydrotherapeutic remedies, which he had come to know from Louis Kuhne. He later claimed to have employed these treatments to cure his wife's hemorrhage, his own pleurisy, and patients who had been affected with the black plague. Gandhi did not

---

6   The following historical description of Gandhi's approach to health is based on his autobiography (2010) [1927], Rothermund (2003), Suhrud (2011), Sarkar (2011), and Brown (1989).

7   According to Alter (2000), Gandhi saw himself as a scientist, drawing on ideas taken from non-compliant medical practitioners in Europe and verifying them on his own body through experiments. Gandhi was thus torn between tradition and modernity, creating something new by the fusion of different elements.

believe in Ayurveda, Siddha or Unani: *"The doctors, vaidyas and hakims have alike failed to enlighten me"* (ibid: 193). This aversion was justified by Gandhi's mistrust of any kind of medication:

> Though I have had two serious illnesses in my life, I believe that man has little need to drug himself. 999 cases out of a thousand can be brought round by means of a well-regulated diet, water and earth treatment and similar household remedies. He who runs to a doctor, *vaidya* or *hakim* for every little ailment, and swallows all kind of vegetable and mineral drugs, not only curtails his life, but, by becoming the slave of his body instead of remaining its master, loses self-control, and ceases to be a man (ibid: 245).

Gandhi disapproved of the way Ayurveda had become institutionalized and therefore absorbed under the colonial regime. Naturopathy was for him the only means of effecting healing within the body, rather than imposing something on the body. Thus, it was the only system striving for prevention and integrating a focus on health into daily life. However, Gandhi directed most of his mistrust towards Allopathy, its doctors and its treatments: he equated being under allopathic treatment with slavery. In the manifesto *Hind Swaraj*, for instance, he explains how a vicious circle of overeating and taking allopathic pills can weaken body and mind:

> I overeat, I have indigestion, I go to a doctor, he gives me medicine, I am cured. I overeat again, I take his pills again. Had I not taken the pills in the first instance I would have suffered the punishment deserved by me and I would not have overeaten again. [...] Had the doctor not intervened, Nature would have done its work and I would have acquired mastery over myself, would have been freed from vice and would have become happy (Gandhi 1909: 3).

In Gandhi's view, the emphasis should lie on a simple lifestyle with local products and food. Nature played a significant role in the description of this lifestyle. He conducted experiments to legitimize his approaches and to give them a scientific slant. He then published the results of these experiments in order to reach a wider audience. Gandhi disapproved not only of allopathic, ayurvedic and other medical practitioners and medication but condemned everything he regarded as a Western, imperial or invasive lifestyle.

Health, Body and Building the Nation

After his return to India, Gandhi became more radical in terms of diet and decided to go for periods completely without food. Gandhi's very special diet, consisting of fruits, nuts and periods of fasting, became part of his philosophy of *satyagraha*, a neologism derived from the Sanskrit word *satya* (truth) and *agraha* (holding, insistence). *Satyagraha* was also meant to describe the movement of civil disobedience, which began in South Africa and finally led India to its independence. For instance, in 1932 Gandhi fasted in order to prevent separate elections for caste-less or untouchables. In prison at the time, he decided to fast to death if necessary to call attention to this issue, and this campaign provoked a strong reaction. His fast was so shocking to the public that decision-makers opted to give untouchables the right to enter temples to which they had formerly been refused access. In the end, the dispute between the British government and Gandhi was settled by the promise of a quota of reserved seats. Thus, the embodied practice of fasting became a strategic political instrument or even a weapon used to express a specific opinion. This method was intended to demonstrate to an adversary the Truth without force, and Gandhi saw it as the last means when all other methods had failed, especially in the context of the battle for independence and building an Indian nation (Trivedi 2007, Alter 2000).

As Gandhi attests in *Key to Health* (1942), his book on medical philosophy (or public health as we would call it nowadays), he had a specific interest in dissemination and increasing the accessibility of the results of his experiments to the public. He wanted to convince the people of the need for self-restraint and self-control over their own bodies:

> The fact remains that the doctors induce us to indulge, and the result is that we have become deprived of self-control and have become effeminate. In these circumstances, we are unfit to serve the country. To study European medicine is to deepen our slavery (Gandhi 1909: 59).

A change in diet and the avoidance of any kind of medication were intended to foster a moral change, a shift towards being more "civilized." Gandhi saw this moral change as a precondition for a powerful and self-determined Indian nation. He did not, of course, equate "civilized" with a superior Western civilization, as the British did. Instead, as he explains in *Hind Sawaraj* (1909), by civilization he meant a way of behavior surrendered to duties and morals, and being the master of one's senses and passions. Gandhi disseminated his idea through several journals, such as *The Indian Opinion* published in South Africa, and wrote several books on health and disease.

Ultimately, his philosophy was formed through a combination of his own experiences, lessons from the Gita in a generic sense, German Naturopaths, Russian philosophers and discussions with fellow countrymen. The result is not only an eclectic and self-contained philosophy – consisting of flows from all over the world – but a concept that has been formed into a complete, contemporary medical system. Ironically, for his *embodiment of resistance* Gandhi drew heavily upon concepts from abroad, including the countries of the colonizers, in order to legitimize his approach.

Other First Generation Naturopaths in South India

Besides the two well-known figures of South Indian Naturopathy mentioned in the introduction, C. R. R. Varma and Ramakrishnan, other channels of knowledge dissemination can be traced. Even before Gandhi's interest in naturopathic treatment methods became famous, in 1894 Dr. Venkat Chelapati Sharma from Andrah Pradesh translated Kuhne's book into Telugo. A few years later, it was translated into Hindi and Urdu. Translations of the writings of other European practitioners followed and Naturopathy suddenly had a great audience among a segment of the population that was increasingly critical of colonial methods of handling public health. These people did not regard Ayurveda as a viable treatment option due to how oppressed its practice and practitioners had become by the colonialists. A whole school of Indian Naturopaths arose. The most prominent among them was Dr. Krishnan Raju, who opened a hospital in Vijayawada, Andrah Pradesh, and Dr. Sitaram Jindal, the founder of the biggest Naturopathy hospital in Asia near Bangalore. Others such as K. Lakshmana Sarma, J.M. Jussawalla, S.J. Singh and S. Swaminathan became famous for their publications on naturopathic treatment methods (see, for example, Sarma and Swaminathan 1993, Singh 1980 and Jussuwalla 1956) and therefore provided the basis for a broader appreciation of Naturopathy as well as the foundation for its professionalization (Jindal 2002, Alter 2000, Kumar 2005, Nair and Nanda 2014).

Although both Swaminathan and Lakshaman Sarma published and practiced in South India, C. R. R. Varma and Ramakrishnan became the point of reference for naturopathic development in this area. They are, of course, only two examples of the historical link between Gandhi and contemporary Naturopathy in India. Ramakrishnan added a very local feature to his practice by saying that *"Coconut and banana are the best food humans can have"* since these are the fruits that call forth sentiments and pride for one's native country or homeland. Both Varma and Ramakrishnan had political intentions: Varma refused to build a hospital or clinic so as to avoid specialization, institutionalization and power hierarchies. Ramakrishnan's focus was oriented towards exposing the hazards of consumption. At the same time, like Gandhi, both of their theories and practices also drew upon and referred to Western ideology and therefore give a glimpse of the heterogeneous interpretations of Gandhi's legacy as well as that of European practitioners. Thus, the following section illustrates how the merger between German Naturopathy and Indian philosophy took shape.

3   Brothers in Arms: German Pioneers

Naturopathic treatment methods were developed in Europe during the 19th century, based on the exclusive use of natural elements to treat illnesses by facilitating the body's ability to heal itself. The explicit use of food for healing purposes played the dominant role. European practitioners developed these treatments as alternatives to increasingly invasive allopathic practices and synthetically-produced drugs. Their common aim, according to Alter (2000), was to have their patients retain power over their own bodies. They believed that knowledge about health and disease should not be monopolized by specialists but should be accessible to the people.

Naturopaths certainly influenced and copied from each other but they still differed in the details of their treatments. At least in the German-speaking area, Naturopaths were strongly influenced by Jean-Jacques Rousseau's philosophy, his concept of nature, vegetarianism, and critique of civilization's process and progress. With the help of treatment methods drawing on the "natural power" of the sun, water and earth, practitioners as laymen tried to help themselves and others. Since nature was pretty bewildering at times, Naturopaths helped to translate. Positive examples of so-called natural behavior were "prehistoric men" or "primitives," healthfully living naked in forests and bearing bad weather conditions as well as any kind of disease. Naturopaths also used the behavior of animals at times as a model for the right way to live (Heyll 2006).

The conception of nature for European Naturopaths in the first half of the 19th century was strongly connected with a romantic image of the forest. German painters – such as Caspar David Friedrich – were known for depicting scenes of uninhabited environments, particularly forests with a single human being, in the process of being confronted by this vast wilderness. The forest is seen as wild and left to its own devices. It is a symbol of primordial and unrestrained forces rather than a frontier in the liberal enlightenment sense. Friedrich's pictures have been interpreted as a prose on native nature, and further, as a critique against the intrusive intervention into nature and especially into the forest as its representative (Wettengl 1990). In the same way as European and Indian Naturopaths of the 21st century, Romantic art celebrates the ideas of homeland in reaction to emerging industrialization and economic modernization, and extols anti-civilization development in society. According to these artists and philosophers, the increasing urbanization and industrialization of society foster a view of nature as purely a resource for human consumption and exploitation. Historians consider this period to be the basis of the ecological movement in Europe (Allard 2007, Löwy 1987, Oerlemans 2002).

Several prominent German Naturopaths deserve mention. As one of the first Naturopaths in the German-speaking area, Vincent Prießnitz (1799-1851) watched a deer curing its wound in a pond and thereafter developed his famous hydro-therapeutic methods with cold water. Johannes Schroth (1789-1856), the founder of the famous Schroth-Cure, was a schoolmate of Prießnitz and experimented with dried bread in order to heal disease. Arnold Rikli (1823-1906), a Swiss Naturopath, is the founder of the atmospheric cure in which he used alternating baths in the sun, water, earth and air for promoting recovery. Most striking about Rikli is that he used these treatments and assigned four elements – water, air, sun and earth – to them in order to give his method of treatment a stronger semblance of nature (Heyll 2006), a formulation that has been influential in contemporary Indian Naturopathy.

Louis Kuhne and the Theory of Toxemia

Louis Kuhne (1835-1901) suffered from diseases that were not cured by allopathic medicine and was in search of alternatives. He was one of the most prominent practitioners to treat disease by enhancing the vital forces of his patients through the consumption of raw, vegetarian food and milk. According to Kuhne, disease is a consequence of toxemia, the poisoning of the body through the non-excretion of harmful materials:

> We now come quite naturally to the definition of disease. Disease is the presence of foreign matters in the system. For the correctness of this definition there is an infallible test. If after that which we have designated as morbid matter has in a suitable manner been removed from the system, the disease itself disappears, and the body at the same time regains its *normal form*, the truth of our definition has been established (Kuhne 2003 [1899]: 19, emphasis by Kuhne).

Since toxemia is considered to be the cause of all diseases, Kuhne claimed: "*It is, therefore, the doctrine of the Unity of Disease which I teach and defend* [...]"

(Kuhne ibid: 28).[8] Healing thus takes place through detoxification and purification of the body. Although diseases are unified under one causal pathway (toxemia), some treatment methods are better for certain diseases than others. This contradiction is common to most naturopathic practitioners of Kuhne's time; however none of them expatiated it to the same extent.

Kuhne introduced hydro-therapeutic treatment methods: fever is diverted through cold baths, rheumatism treated with steam baths, whooping cough with diverting baths. Kuhne provided detailed illustrations about the construction of steam baths and full steam baths. He also developed a facial diagnostic method, a technique that is well-received and much discussed in India but in fact was never implemented. Kuhne disapproved of allopathic medication or surgery. In his seminal work *New Science of Healing*, originally published in 1899, Kuhne developed an anti-civilization critique of 19th century German society. He argued that the modern lifestyle of the European fin-de-ciècle – characterized by urbanization and industrialization – alienates humans and animals from their natural behavior, which accordingly has a strong impact on their health. For instance, he described the emergence of new diseases in animals caused by artificially living in the company of humans. Similarly, humans become ill when they deviate from their natural food sources and ways of life. Kuhne contrasted this world of urbanization and industrialization with the idealized image of the original state he detected in nature, a concept very much informed by Romanticism and Rousseau. In 1883, Kuhne opened his own sanatorium close to Leipzig, where he attempted to combine simplicity with efficacy in treatments.

Another pioneer, John Tildon (1851-1940) from Illinois, USA, took up Kuhne's theory of the unity of disease and rendered it more specific. According to him, toxemia is the fundamental causal factor for all disease. It is caused by overeating or eating the wrong food. The concept of "enervation" plays a major role: enervation is the lack of power to fight accumulating toxins (Singh 1980).

Just's and Kneipp's Methods of Treatment

Adolf Just (1859-1936) had a similar approach. Suffering from enervation, he adopted Prießnitz's, Kneipp's and also Samuel Hahnemann's methods in order to find a cure for his own medical condition. Just is especially famous for the use of mud packs and baths, but only those using cold water since "*on the whole, of the warming of the water; it is against nature*" (Just 1903 available at Just 1996: 29). In his publication *Return to Nature* (ibid), he explains the effect and handling of mud packs and hydrotherapy. Most striking about Just's

---

8   As a mnemonic this sentence is also emphasized in the original version by the author.

approach is his radical rejection of processed food, allopathic medicine and any kind of science, even diagnostics and examinations. In his view, the body has the ability to heal all diseases by itself, aided only by adapting one's lifestyle to nature. Therefore any kind of additional exercise is unnecessary in the healing process. In 1886, Just's hospital, named Jungborn ("born young"), opened in eastern Germany next to the Hartz Mountains and attracted quite a crowd of stakeholders interested in alternative medicine. Since Gandhi was especially interested in Just's methods, he even sent a delegate to visit.[9]

Sebastian Kneipp (1821-1897) was a Bavarian priest who suffered from tuberculosis during his theology studies. Influenced by the reading of Prießnitz, Kneipp cured himself with the ice-cold water of the Danube River. Despite criticism, Kneipp's treatments became famous in the era of cholera and attracted an increasing number of followers. In the 1860s and 1870s several bath houses opened in Bad Wörishofen and its surroundings that were dedicated to offering these services. Kneipp published *My Water-Cure* in 1886 explaining his hydrotherapy treatments, which consisted of ablutions, vapors, shower baths, water wading and bandages. Nowadays his ideas are subsumed in a five pillar principle: Water, plants, exercise, nutrition and balance. Water is involved in all the above-mentioned forms of hydro-therapeutic treatment. Plants are used in herbal treatments such as packs or by direct consumption. Kneipp integrated exercise such as water wading into hydrotherapeutic treatments, but compared to other, more radical Naturopaths, he was only minimally concerned about exercise. In contrast, he dealt with the topic of nutrition in great detail: Kneipp had very specific ideas about the effect of particular foodstuffs; although his conceptualization did not insist on vegetarian food, he basically recommended a balanced diet. The fifth pillar ascribed to Kneipp is balance, which serves as the organizing principle or organizing theory for the four others, as people say in *Kneipp Bund*[10] and hospitals. A U.S. website, promoting Kneipp's ideas, concepts and most of all cosmetic products, describes this fifth pillar as follows:

---

9   The Jungborn hospital fell victim to ww2 but was rebuilt later on. More information on the visit of Gandhi's delegate can be found at Internet source Jungborn 2016.

10   The *Kneipp Bund* is an alliance of practitioners in Germany that has several branches. It grants licenses to practice the therapies. The alliance offers further training, organizes research, negotiates with health insurance providers and controls the quality and standard of treatment in their associated centers. For further information see Internet source Kneippbund 2016 (in German). According to their Journal, it was only in 1980 that representatives of different Kneipp Associations adopted the "Principles for Physiotherapy according to Kneipp" and the theory of the five pillars emerged (Kneipp-Journal 2010:188).

> Balance: A balanced lifestyle – the basis for a healthy, active, and satisfying life. Water, plants, exercise, and nutrition: Each of these elements contributes uniquely to your health and enjoyment of life. Yet, according to Sebastian Kneipp, it is the interaction of all four elements that keeps the body and spirit in equilibrium (Internet source Kneipp 2016).

The rather indefinite nature of this fifth pillar is constituted by its umbrella function: Balance integrates all four principles and gives them equal validation. However, balance also possesses the extra meanings of psychological equilibrium, stress tolerance and even social competence. In order to gain more spiritual maturity, practitioners of Kneipp institutions nowadays resort to treatments such as Yoga, progressive muscle-relaxation or Tai Chi (Internet source Kneippbund 2016, Uehleke and Hentschel 2006). The Naturopath Benedict Lust (1872-1945) was strongly influenced by Kneipp's theories after being cured of tuberculosis. Lust emigrated to the USA and opened several institutions in order to promote Naturopathy.

Kneipp, Kuhne and Just all opened highly-frequented sanatoriums, which still exist today and are booming due to a high demand and clever marketing strategies. The promotion of health and healthy living beyond merely curing disease is a common motif for all naturopathic institutions. Most striking about them is the fact that none of these practitioners had an allopathic education; they were laymen doctors convinced by the ideology behind Naturopathy. Only Kneipp sought to interact with allopathic practitioners, and for this he was accused of major betrayal (Heyll 2006).

Of course, this German trio only represents a few of the many influential Naturopaths in the United States and other European countries. Still, when talking about the origins of Naturopathy in India, these three and their above-mentioned ideas and concepts have been referred to most often. Indian educational books as well as patients have cited Kneipp, Kuhne and Just.

Naturopaths from central Europe, some explicitly such as Rikli but most implicitly such as Just, have used the ancient Greek idea of four elements (water, earth, sun and air), deeply rooted in European philosophy, in order to organize their treatments. They assigned local hydrotherapeutic treatments, steam baths, full body baths and the drinking of fluids to the element of water; earth treatments such as packs, baths, scrubs and also the metaphysical connection between people and their land to the element of earth; and any kind of movement outside, the intake of sun or air by exposure of the body, or simply breathing, to the elements of sun or air. Diet is an additional factor common to all Naturopaths and is generally attributed great importance. Although the approach varies, some Naturopaths recommend living on a raw diet, some even recommend regular fasting and others prefers a "light" diet. Overall, European Naturopaths consider Naturopathy, its ideology and its treatments to be part of a critique on civilization, on the increasingly invasive methods of Allopathy and on the exploitation of industrialization, where people have ceased to have choices in their lives and therefore are unable to be the masters of their own bodies.

There are strong similarities between the approaches that drove Gandhi and European naturopathic practitioners. Gandhi appropriated hydrotherapeutic and mud applications from practitioners such as Kuhne, Kneipp and Just. Similarly, he developed a conception of nature that relied upon the ideas of European practitioners in the first half of the 19th century. For him, naturopathic treatments were a similar form of resistance against hegemonic political circumstances. The idea of building a nation through moralizing its people is unique to Gandhi's approach. Gandhi used related categories of elements from Rikli's approach to organize treatment modalities.

4   Yoga as the Fifth Element? Contemporary Adaptations

In India today, Naturopathy is organized according to the *panchabutha* system, by the five elements of ether, air, fire, water and earth. These elements were first mentioned in the *vedas*, more precisely the *Rigveda*.[11] It was Gandhi who initially brought Rikli's categorization of four elements into connection with Naturopathy by writing:

> The world is compounded of the five elements – earth, water, air, fire, and ether. So too is our body. It is a sort of miniature world. Hence the body stands in need of all these elements in due proportion, pure earth. Pure water, pure fire or sunlight, pure air, and open space. When any one of these falls short of its due proportion, illness is caused in the body (Gandhi 1921: 11).

In the subsequent passages of the book, Gandhi referred to air and water treatments, and the right way to live in terms of diet, exercise, attire and sexual relationships. Although his classification of treatments and elements is not consistent through all five elements, Gandhi certainly provided a starting point for naturopathic theory in India.

---

11   See, for example, a summary of the *Rigvedas* in Mittal (2005: 45ff.).

According to Alter (2000, 2011), the adaptation of five elements and the combination of naturopathic treatments with Yoga perfectly reflects the latter's nature and its strong similarity to naturopathic ideology. Alter argues that the promotion of Yoga as an activity to boost health is a new development, fostered by pioneers such as Shri Yogendra, who opened the first Yoga Institute in New York and later another one in Bombay. He thereby propagated the idea of Yoga as a treatment for specific diseases and personal hygiene. Shri Yogendra had many followers in India and abroad, and a great interest in "Eastern practices" led Yoga to become popular in the Indian as well as the Western middle class. Alter describes another dimension of Yoga, where it became an integral part of the politics of *swadeshi* (self-sufficiency) and a symbol of India's national identity and sophistication. Yoga promoters started to use the language of biomedicine in order to be understood by a larger audience and to clarify the efficacy of yogic treatments. In this sense, Naturopathy and Yoga were consolidated *"in terms of a new language of science being articulated against two forms of hegemony, one political, economic and geographical, the other medical and ideological"* (Alter 2000: 69). Alter argues further that Yoga was easily introduced into this new naturopathic philosophy because it could occupy the fifth element, non-existent in European Naturopathy: ether. Although this seems to be logical, in naturopathic college education, Yoga does not constitute the element of ether, and it is subsumed along with others under the element air.

According to a text book written by Rakesh Jindal (2002), the five elements can be hierarchized as follows: Ether is the most subtle, followed by air, fire and water, while earth has the most physical manifestation. Treatments differ according to the element that is being targeted. For instance, the treatment assigned to the element ether includes celibacy, self-control, resting, and relaxation through fasting and meditation. Gandhi's philosophy of *Satyagraha* is mentioned as a reference in conjunction with this (ibid: 77-96). Air-related treatments are, of course, mainly breathing fresh air, air baths, breathing exercises such as *pranayamas*, but also massages and everything related to movement. Therefore gymnastics and sports such as swimming and horseback riding are recommended in the book as well as Yoga postures. These Yoga *asanas* are strictly categorized by their efficacy in combating specific health conditions (ibid: 97-138). Treatments ascribed to the element of sun consist, for example, of light treatments. The idea that rays of colored light have the power to influence mood and to relieve pain is common even in an allopathic context. In Naturopathy this concept is extended by the attribution of diseases to seven colors, fractured in a prism. Additionally, Jindal explains sun baths with and without a water element, for instance wet clothes, the consumption of hot water or variations in the temperature of baths (ibid: 140-158). Water treatments feature adaptations of Kuhne's, Kneipp's and Just's proposals: Hip baths, spinal baths, full body baths and wet bandages, as well as drinking water and enemas. Jindal also describes stomach baths, a cleansing process of the stomach through vomiting salt water (ibid: 159-174). Treatments assigned to the element earth include mud baths and mud bandages, traditions influenced by Just (ibid: 177-182). All element-related treatments are supported by sections of the *vedas*, which Jindal cites to substantiate a treatment logic based on the five elements. Diet is an additional component in the treatment of all diseases and is discussed at length by Jindal. With reference to nutritional science, he describes the perfect constitution of a balanced diet, and explains the use of proteins, fats, minerals, carbohydrates and vitamins.

The contemporary Indian philosophy of Naturopathy draws upon Kuhne's theory about unity of disease, and Tildon's concept of enervation. A drawing of the toxemia tree (Figure 2),[12] found in many Indian textbooks on Naturopathy, confirms this strong dependence on Tildon and Kuhne:

As Figure 2 shows, diseases are rooted in an incorrect lifestyle such as bad nutrition, medication or overeating. These erroneous food habits lead to enervation, and enervation is the cause of all diseases, as illustrated in the branches of the tree. Since the diseases in the branches have a modern description (such as HIV), the tree is not a creation of Tildon or his contemporaries but rather is an illustration produced by Indian Naturopaths in recent decades.

According to this theory, diagnosis is unnecessary because the roots of all diseases are seen to be the same. However, textbooks such as Jindal's enumerate and anatomize a great number of diseases and explain in detail their preferable naturopathic treatment. This contradiction is evident throughout the history of Naturopathy.

The contemporary classification of naturopathic treatments can be traced as follows: European practitioners such as Kuhne and Rikli differentiated naturopathic treatments according to four elements: water, earth, sun and light. Gandhi built on and "Indianized" the categorization of treatments by adding a fifth element. However, he focused on treatments using the elements of water and air while also discussing questions concerning food. Other Indian pioneers of Naturopathy such as Jindal modified this system and systematically ascribed treatments to all five elements. These treatments refer to naturopathic textbooks. They consisted of Yoga as a healing system and other non-medicinal treatments (e.g. healing through colors). Furthermore, some aspects of ayurvedic treatments were integrated, such as cleansing the stomach through

---

12   Nisargopachar 2009a: 24

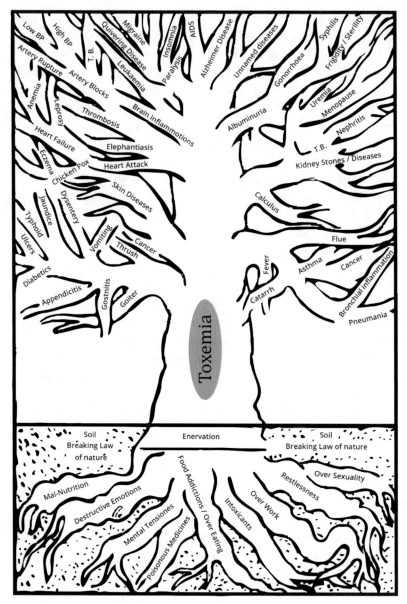

FIGURE 2   *"Detoxify for Health"*

vomiting. Since Yoga also relies on the *panchabutha* element structure, strong theoretical similarities made its integration with Naturopathy quite easy, if not to say natural. As Alter (2000) notes, Benedict Lust already attended Yoga lectures in the United States and India in the early 1930s, and articles were published about the need for syntheses between Yoga and Naturopathy. Yoga is an important aspect of the whole system. The specific concept of nature within Indian naturopathic textbooks is based on European Romanticism, Rousseau and other proponents of the Enlightenment. Therefore it is no surprise that the slogan "living like animals in the forest" became the superior goal of naturopathic ideology in South India.

5   Conclusion

Provoked by the systematic oppression of so-called indigenous medicine (such as Ayurveda and Unani) during colonialism, the political activist Gandhi resisted the economic and political occupation and exploitation of his country. He also rebelled against the coercion of using an imposed medical system that felt cruel and invasive to him and many others. He therefore used treatment methods (such as medical flows) imported from Europe and merged them with local ideas in order to create a new health system, one that was compatible with his non-violent philosophy.

The aim of this chapter was to trace the logic of naturopathic theory and treatment methods in a historical context. Gandhi, Just, Kuhne, Kneipp, Varma and Ramakrishnan embraced different approaches and placed different emphases in Naturopathy: Gandhi used naturopathic treatments as a political instrument, Kuhne provided a structural theory of etiology, Just and Kneipp experimented with water and earth treatments, Varma wanted to educate his people in Kerala about health and disease and thereby empower them, and radical experimenter Ramakrishnan even sacrificed his life through his condemnation of consumption.

To summarize, when speaking of the history of Naturopathy from Central Europe to India, certain similarities are evident. First, the lifestyle of the practitioners greatly influenced their practices: Most of the practitioners started treating themselves with naturopathic methods because of the ineffectiveness of Allopathy. Thereafter they changed their living habits according to what they felt to be "in tune with nature." Second, their diet consisted of local and preferably raw or unprocessed produce. Even if diet was not integrated in a theoretical context – for instance the categorization of the *panchabutha* system – it was given special attention. Third, while the theory of Naturopathy is easy to grasp due to its few basic principles, the actual treatment methods can differ enormously. Practitioners use the language of allopathic science, as well as its understandings of etiology and anatomy, in order to legitimize and implement their practice. The overall aim was, and continues to be for many adherents, a critique of social conditions expressed through the *embodiment of resistance*. Practitioners employed naturopathic treatment methods in a bid to free themselves and others from imperialism. Thus, the body has been the instrument to express this resistance.

PART 2

Naturopathy in Practice

∵

Introduction to Part 2

In theory Naturopathy is designed as a self-contained medical system, one among many institutionalized and non-institutionalized systems in India's pluralistic medical landscape. However, it holds a special position because of its specific characteristics. In *Yoga in Modern India* (2004), the anthropologist Joseph Alter argues that Naturopathy in India does not follow the concept of a clinic in a Foucauldian sense. Rather, naturopathic practices can be better grasped as an anti-clinic, acting subversively in relation to hegemonic medical systems. Alter argues that Naturopathy *"can pose a serious challenge to medicine's modernity by destabilizing the structure of biopower upon which postcolonial governmentality is based"* (Alter 2004: 112).

First, integral to medicine's modernity – in other words, the clinic – is the possibility of medical investigations through the categorization of patients according to symptoms and disease development, or the probability and frequency of patients' etiopathogenesis. The second characteristic of the modern clinic relates to the clinical gaze as a new epistemological approach to handling patients. The clinical gaze refers to the dehumanizing medical separation of the patient's body from the patient's identity or whole person (Foucault 1973). For Foucault, the concept of power plays a major role. The institutionalization of medicine and the respective construction of specialist knowledge – dovetailing with power in a functional manner – result in the establishment of a (medical) norm, against which individual health can be measured. Technologies of discipline guarantee repression by fostering new effectiveness of power through control, verification and normalizing sanctions. Hospitals as institutions establish a network of surveillance over the human body, which leads to the internalization of these expectations and therefore to a self-observing, self-monitoring individual (Foucault 1977, Seier 2001, Dreyfus and Rabinow 1984, Jaye et al. 2006, Samuelsen and Steffen 2004).

The above discussion is relevant to the remaining chapters of this book in a number of ways. First, I aim to acknowledge and differentiate between several approaches of contemporary Naturopaths in India – an endeavor I undertake by examining the two most prominent branches in South India, *professionals* and *psycho-nutritionals*. I explore how Naturopaths conceive of and treat the human body, and how their approach correlates with the Foucauldian notion of the clinical gaze. Central to this discussion is the matter of power asymmetries. The anti-clinic changes the relationship of the doctor to the patient insofar as agency is transferred from the former to the latter by suspending the imbalance in knowledge. The patient in the clinic is a passive object, committed to the judgment of the emerged professionalized physician and subject to the biopolitics of governmental institutions. Therefore, in theory, the patient of the anti-clinic is responsible, active and informed. Thus, the second section of this book is about the organization of naturopathic treatment centers and how the doctor-patient relationship plays out in the ideology and social practice of Naturopathy in South India.

CHAPTER 3

Evidence versus Experience: Two Streams of Naturopathy in South India

Contemporary Indian naturopaths refer to a very small pool of literature, thereby establishing a coherent system of self-contained healing theory. The use of just a few pioneer texts written by Gandhi, Kuhne and Varma appears to be instrumental to maintaining an external image of homogeneity. This is in line with Naturopaths' oral construction of the historic evolution of Naturopathy in Europe and its integration into the *panchabutha* Weltanschauung, i.e. the five elements of the *vedas* that build the ontological basis of existence. At first glance this seems to contradict Sujatha's findings in her ethnography of Siddha in India (2007), which pointed towards structural pluralism implying heterogeneity and multiplicity of layers and genres within all systems of medicine. However, to social scientists in general and medical anthropologists in particular, a divergence between theoretical healing concepts and their implementation in local socio-medical practices is empirically evident (Horden 2013). Often the interpretation of healing theory is a major tool of delineation into separate groups (Mol 2008). In the context of contemporary South Indian Naturopathy there are two main readings of Kuhne, Kneipp, Gandhi, Varma and others that indeed are used to constitute two diverging vocational streams of healing: the professionals and the psycho-nutritionals. This chapter is engaged with the configuration of these two interpretations of naturopathic theory in India.

Professionals remain cohesive predominantly as a result of their institutions; their development and collaboration will therefore be the focus of the first part of this chapter. The second most striking feature about professionals is their standardization of practice, which has been a result of the standardization of education. Professionalization is taking place on a national level and will therefore be examined as such.[1]

The second part of the chapter presents the ideology of the more local South Indian stream of naturopathic practitioners: Psycho-nutritionals. With the aid

---

[1] In the 1970s, Leslie (1972) and Brass (1973) documented a general tendency towards professionalization within all of the Indian systems of medicine such as Ayurveda or Unani. Professionalization has certainly intensified the contemporary practice of these systems. However, as Trawick (1991) shows, there are still examples of ethnographic work on non-scholarly-trained *vaidyas*.

of three analytical categories (contesting globalization and Western civilization, simplicity and transparency, and empowerment), the characteristics of psycho-nutritionals are discussed and contrasted with the practice of professionals. The phenomenon of two medical branches relying on the same European imports combined with "Indian elements," but differing in many aspects such as their aims and goals, is quite unique among medical systems in India.

In Kerala, the dispute and battle over interpretative power between professionals and psycho-nutritionals has grown more acute with the introduction of legal registration. The development and outcome of this dispute is the focus of the last section of the chapter. The tension is not only concerned with medical discourse, but rather it reflects a contest over who holds legitimate rights to represent "true" Indian Naturopathy both to the outside and the inside. In Kerala, both sides see themselves as representing contemporary Naturopathy practice. This current struggle for interpretative authority is also, of course, one of access to resources – public and private – that will significantly influence the predominance of medical practices in the field.

1   Science in the Making

The first group of Naturopaths constitutes a highly professionalized segment of the medical system in India. Its most distinguishing characteristics are its institutions and patterns of education, both of which demonstrate professionals' increasing institutionalization and standardization.

Just as it is for all medical systems under AYUSH, there are different bodies that support the systems of Naturopathy and Yoga in India: The National Institute of Naturopathy (NIN)[2] located in Pune, the Yogic equivalent Morarji Desai National Institute of Yoga (MDNIY)[3] located in Delhi, and the research body, the Central Council for Research in Yoga and Naturopathy (CCRYN),[4] likewise located in Delhi. Their relationship to each other is depicted in Figure 3.

AYUSH funds all three institutions. CCRYN is connected to each of the other institutions in order to enhance research activities, share data and disseminate information relating to the standardization of naturopathic practice.

---

2   NIN 2015

3   MDNIY 2015

4   CCRYN 2015

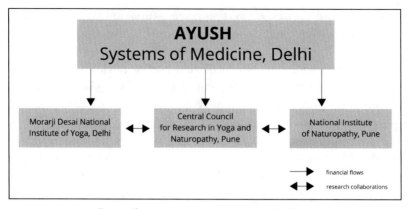

FIGURE 3   *Constellation of government institutions related to Naturopathy*

The Central Council for Research in Yoga and Naturopathy (CCRYN) can be found in the same building as the headquarters of AYUSH in Delhi, together with the research bodies of the other medical systems. Their main aim is to fund and support diverse research activities nationwide. Surprisingly, out of the 30 research projects conducted so far, none have been conducted using Naturopathy alone. If research has been carried out into naturopathic methods, it has always been in conjunction with some type of Yogic treatment. On the other hand, scientific studies have been conducted into Yoga in comparison to other medical systems, since double-blind studies in Yoga are impossible. Studies that include Naturopathy to varying degrees have only been published with general information about the system of Naturopathy and research methodology, where students learn how to draw up clinical trials and implement the methodology for clinical research. The employees of CCRYN are open to any kind of research application, but since a PhD has not yet been launched in Naturopathy, it will apparently take some more time until this kind of research is established and published on a broader level. CCRYN is currently running eight outpatient departments, primarily in Delhi. CCRYN also publishes a quarterly magazine named *Yogic Pracritic Jeevan*, which provides an overview of the activities and campaigns undertaken by CCRYN. According to the magazine, they have a constant stream of publications, literature and clinical research.[5]

The National Institute of Naturopathy (NIN) was founded in 1986 in Pune on a historical site, as employees like to tell visitors: the location of a sanatorium frequently visited by Mahatma Gandhi. It is close to the railway station and is

---

5   This information was provided by Surender Sandhu, an employee of CCRYN.

therefore central but on a quiet side street. Apart from the main building containing offices and a huge library, there are treatment buildings for men and women, a Yoga hall, a shop stocked with health-related articles and publications, a praying hall in which a small corner is decorated with Mahatma Gandhi souvenirs, a huge garden, and a diet corner (or dining room) offering "natural food." This diet corner is public and also serves as a popular restaurant for local business people on their lunch breaks. The staff consists of ten doctors who are supported by interns from the college of Naturopathy. At the moment the NIN is an outpatient hospital, which keeps the campus bustling with visitors on a daily basis. Patients can either pay for each single treatment or they can buy monthly packages. In the evenings one can attend lectures about specific diseases and their treatment; the latter are open to the public but are attended mostly by employees. Most recently, the first course on research methodology in Naturopathy for BNYS students commenced. In addition, a one-year training course is on offer to treatment attendants, employees specifically trained to carry out therapies.

The former head of the department, Dr. Babu Joseph, plans to open an affiliated college near the center in order to foster a more fruitful combination of education and practice. He is very concerned about enhancing the research abilities of BNYS doctors. In his opinion, research should be the main focus of Naturopathy in the near future:

> Unless your system is a documented system, an evidence-based system, the world is not going to accept it on scientific terms, so for the acceptance of the scientific world you have to make any system an evidence-based system.

NIN provides financial support for one-day or five-day health camps in about 500 different naturopathic institutions all over India. In order to receive funding from the NIN, the institutions have to apply, follow the guidelines – thereby proving their professionalism – and submit a detailed report afterwards. Through these requirements, Dr. Babu Joseph and his employees are trying to establish a standard for naturopathic activities throughout all of the affiliated institutions. NIN publishes a bilingual magazine called *Nisargopachar* in English and Hindi. Every month the headline is another major topic, such as a disease or a current event. Various authors from inside and outside the institution review books and articles and answer questions about specific diseases in a very practical manner. The ideology undergirding professionalized Naturopathy is evident in two examples from the Question and Answer section of this magazine. In August 2010, the topic of *Nisargopachar* was "Age Old

Problems" (i.e., problems that come with age). In the Question and Answer section, a Mr. Ramesh wrote in to seek help for the following problem:

> My mother has been suffering from asthma for more than 30 years. Nowadays, due to climate changes, she feels flumes in her tongue. Kindly advise the Naturopathy treatments and type of diet to be followed (Nisargopacher 2010a: 12).

Dr. D. Sathyanath, a regular doctor at NIN, provides a two-step answer. He counsels Mr. Ramesh to educate his mother – but more specifically, he advises him to educate her in an allopathic sense. He goes on to explain asthma in allopathic terms:

> Asthma is a long-lasting (chronic) disease of the respiratory system. It is a two-pronged disease. First, inflammation in tubes that carry air to the lungs (bronchial tubes) narrows the airway channels to make breathing difficult [...] (ibid).

Secondly, Dr. Sathyanath advises naturopathic treatment. In this case, he recommends three types of therapies: Eliminative therapies (enemas and fasting), smoothing therapies (hydrotherapy), and constructive therapies (massage and Yoga).

A similar approach can be found in the February 2010 issue in which the main topic is "B. Tech (Health)." Here, Shri Sami Rahmanzai, living in Kabul, Afghanistan, suffers from irritable bowel syndrome and is seeking a naturopathic cure after years of unsuccessful allopathic treatment. Again it is Dr. Sathyanath who explains the signs, symptoms and other impacts of irritable bowel syndrome from an allopathic perspective: He enumerates the symptoms, etiological pathways such as stress, certain foods, and menstrual periods, and claims that "*IBS may be caused by a bacterial infection in the gastrointestinal tract*" (Nisargopachar 2010b: 14). As treatment he recommends fasting, a low-fat diet, hydrotherapy and Yoga. Dr. Sathyanath does not integrate Mr. Rahmanzai's problem into a broader naturopathic context; instead, he prefers to educate him about the allopathic-based etiology of the diagnosis, including biochemical and physiological reasons, and recommends only naturopathic treatments.

These responses clearly illustrate the politics of NIN: First and foremost, the importance of patient education ("*a proper understanding of the condition*" 2010a, Dr. D. Sathyanath) is evident. This information is provided solely from an allopathic perspective. Up until this point there is no great difference from health magazines provided by allopathic publishers. It is only the treatment that varies significantly: The idea of using eliminative therapy demonstrates that the underlying concept is the idea of a contaminated body that has to be purged. The other therapies, as Dr. D. Sathyanath maintains, are specifically naturopathic. NIN aims to train its audience in the transparency of a disease and in self-help.

NIN provides information through its magazines, training, funding of camps, and lectures in order to educate the public (and of course their own affiliates). This education is strongly based on allopathic categories, predominantly when it comes to explaining the diseases. As Dr. Babu Joseph emphasized, adapting allopathic vocabulary is the only way to even be considered in the limited circle of evidence-based medicine in India. This is also the normative standard they set towards affiliated and subordinated hospitals throughout India. As Lambert (2009) points out, this *"evidence of effectiveness"* by means of *"appraising quantitative data of treatment outcomes through the mechanisms of 'systematic review' [...] and 'meta analysis"'* has its roots in the health research and policy of the late 1980s in Western countries. Engler (2003) defines *"scientification"* in the narrow sense of *"materialism, empirical observation, falsification of theories, quantification, a developed conception of proof."* Those factors are all provided by the NIN, who sets the standard. Therefore scientification can be seen as another global flow, appropriated by professionalized Naturopaths in India.

The Morarji Desai National Institute of Yoga (MDNIY) has a central location in Delhi. An equivalent to the NIN in Pune, the MDNIY is the Institute for the *"planning, training, promotion and coordination of Yoga Education, Training, Therapy and Research in all aspects"* (MDNIY 2016). MDNIY has a similar scope as its counterpart NIN and offers a Diploma in Yoga Science, further training for AYUSH and allopathic doctors, and Yoga courses both for specific diseases as well as for the general well-being of outpatients. It also supports research on Yoga. The MDNIY publishes a quarterly journal called *Yoga Vijnana* with the goal of keeping their audience up-to-date about current events.

Thus, together these three institutions set the standards for Naturopathy throughout India: AYUSH functions to bring about official legalization; CCRYN creates campaigns to promote naturopathic research nationwide in India; and NIN provides funding, policy-making initiatives and awareness-raising campaigns through health camps and other work in local Naturopathy hospitals. However, these standards are not yet solidified in comparison to other medical sciences (such as Ayurveda or Allopathy). The research designs and results of naturopathic studies are only published through in-house magazines and books and have not yet been submitted to national and international medical journals.

One more institution deserves mention, since it operates primarily in South India and has gained in popularity in recent years. The Indian Naturopathy and Yoga Graduate Medical Association (INYGMA),[6] founded by young professional scholars in the very south of India, constitutes an example of a local, politicized association whose members strive for stronger regulation by the government in order to distinguish themselves from non-college-educated Naturopaths. Naturopathic practitioners unified by INYGMA are building a network through regular conferences and publications. They seek to establish a platform for continual naturopathic research in order to be accepted in the range of evidence-based medicine currently being practiced. INYGMA is most important in the context of the political struggle to legitimize Naturopathy in South India. With regard to legal registration, discussed later in this chapter, INYGMA is the authority representing college-educated naturopathic practitioners. The development and success of INYGMA is testament to the current lack of credibility bestowed upon government-level decision-making by professionals.

Education

Education in Naturopathy, the state-approved and standardized BNYS (Bachelor of Naturopathy and Yogic Science), is a new and up-and-coming field. The landscape of education in most of the medical fields in India is quite heterogeneous. The parallel existence of both private and government educational institutions, with different program durations and varying priorities, is commonplace. The field of Naturopathy in India is organized in the same manner. AYUSH currently recognizes twelve degree colleges in India, nine of them in South Indian states (but none in Kerala), one in Chattisgargh, one in Madhya Pradesh and one in Gujarat. Two of these colleges are government-operated, while the remaining ones are private. The first one was founded in 1970 in Hyderabad, when a Diploma course was transformed into a Bachelors program to make it equivalent in duration to an allopathic course.[7] To be accepted into

---

6 Internet source INYGMA 2015.

7 In addition, there are an unknown number of courses awarding different kinds of certifications, such as the All India Nature Cure Federation in Delhi (All India Nature Cure Federation 2015). This organization offers a Diploma course in Naturopathy and Yoga, which takes place for two hours every Sunday for 3 months. Another course held in Kottayam, Kerala at the Mahatma Gandhi University lasts six months and leads to a DNYT (Diploma of Naturopathic

TABLE 1 *Syllabus of the five-year* BNYS *course (Duration: 4 years + 1 year Internship): Subjects and teaching hours*

Sl. no.	Subjects	Theory	Practicals and seminar classes	Total hours
Year I BNYS				
1	Anatomy	175	150	325
2	Physiology	175	125	300
3	Biochemistry	100	50	150
4	Philosophy of Nature Cure	200	75	275
5	Yoga Practicals (Non-Exam)	25	150	175
	Total hours	675	550	1225
Year II BNYS				
1	Pathology	200	100	300
2	Microbiology	100	50	150
3	Community Medicine	100	50	150
4	Yoga Philosophy	200	175	375
5	Magnetotherapy and Chromopathy	125	75	200
6	Medical Jurisprudence and Forensic Medicine (Non-Exam)	30	20	50
	Total hours	755	470	1225
Year III BNYS				
1	Manipulative Therapies (Massage, Reflexology, Chiropractice, Osteopathy)	100	100	200
2	Acupuncture	100	75	175
3	Yoga and Physical Culture	150	175	325
4	Fasting Therapy	100	25	125
5	Naturopathy Diagnostics (Facial Diagnosis and Iris Diagnosis)	100	100	200
6	Modern Diagnosis and First Aid	100	100	200
	Total Hours	650	575	1225

TABLE 1   *Syllabus of the five-year BNYS course* (cont.)

Sl. no.	Subjects	Theory	Practicals and seminar classes	Total hours
Year IV BNYS				
1	Dietetics, Nutrition and Herbs	250	100	350
2	Obstetrics and Gynecology	100	50	150
3	Yogic Therapy	150	150	300
4	Hydrotherapy	200	100	300
5	Physiotherapy	200	100	300
	Total Hours	900	500	1400

the Bachelor of Naturopathy and Yogic Science course, one must have finished "plus two" (12 years of school in India) and have qualified in the All India Pre Medical Test (AIPMT).

The duration of the BNYS course at naturopathic colleges ranges from 4 to 4.5 years, depending on the program, plus one year of internship at either the affiliated college or another naturopathic institution.[8] Table 1 depicts an example of a syllabus in brief.

Although the syllabi of the colleges all vary slightly, there is a general movement towards standardization: Dr. Babu Joseph from NIN engages in the progress and unification of all colleges in regular meetings. This is evident in the way the aims and objectives are declared at the very beginning of one of the syllabi:

> The course is aimed at overcoming the lack of properly trained personnel in the field of Naturopathy and Yoga Sciences experienced at present and to fulfill the need of therapists in Yoga and Nature Cure with a proper

---

and Yogic Therapy). However, at the moment its continuation is being reconsidered. Not far from there, in Ottapalam, Pallakad district, Kerala a 3.5 year course will lead to a degree. These are just three examples of the degree "jungle" within naturopathic education. However, I will concentrate only on the BNYS certificate, since it is the only indisputably legally-accepted degree in Naturopathy.

8   The following information comes from the S.D.M. College of Naturopathy and Yogic Sciences in Ujire, Karnataka (Rajiv Gandhi University 2011) and from the J.S.S. College of Naturopathy and Yogic Science, which recently moved to the neighborhood of Coimbatore (Tamil Nadu Dr. M.G.R. Medical University 2005).

scientific background in sufficient numbers (Tamil Nadu Dr. M.G.R. Medical University 2005: 1).

The syllabi of Naturopathy colleges resemble to a great extent the syllabi of allopathic medical colleges. Subjects that are also taught in allopathic colleges (such as anatomy, gynecology, pathology, forensic medicine, and toxicology) account for about 35% of the overall workload, while subjects that are specific to nature cures (such as the philosophy of Yoga, fasting and diet therapy or magnetotherapy) account for the remaining 65%. At the beginning of the studies, allopathic subjects predominate while towards the end of the degree course they are almost phased out. Gandhi's theoretical works are taught in class as well as applications designed by German and Indian pioneers. Most of the naturopathic colleges own laboratories with modern high-tech machines and a well-stocked library. The students in the colleges wear white lab coats and frequently, when visiting an affiliated hospital, stethoscopes around their neck.[9]

The BNYS program focuses on the allopathic view of the body: Explanations of health and disease include biochemical and physiological reasons, and Koch's theories of bacteria and the separation of organs, bones and other parts of the body that can be attacked by disease. However, the key difference between the subject matter of allopathic colleges and naturopathic colleges is the fact that naturopathic healing is not achieved through medication or the use of pharmaceutical products. Instead, naturopathic colleges teach so-called holistic methods for the healing process. This perspective is gaining in popularity: there are plans to open more naturopathic colleges throughout India. This boom can be traced first to the demand of students who want to study Naturopathy in colleges. Secondly, this trend is due to an increasing market for non-allopathic healing methods.

Professional Naturopaths have become institutionalized in their education and networks. The constant production of specialist knowledge, the delineation of lay practitioners and the wholesale appropriation of the institutional and educational structures of Allopathy point to the characteristics of Foucault's clinic. The priority given to evidence-based medicine and therefore the *"evidence of effectiveness"* (Lambert 2009) as a manifested goal further

---

9   Naraindas (2006) gives insight into the syllabi of ayurvedic colleges and describes a related eclectic approach in their education. According to him, ayurvedic colleges have a similar structure: Students are schooled in the basics of (allopathic) anatomy and chemistry as well as in ayurvedic pathogenesis. However, the healing part of their education is concerned with ayuvedic methods.

conforms to Foucault's definition of a clinic. The adaptation of allopathic categories in the conception of the body and the location of disease in the latter indicates the development of a clinical gaze. All these characteristics give reason to the argument that professionalized Naturopathy is in fact not an anti-clinic, creating a different standard for normality, but rather an adaptation of the inherent rules of the clinic. However, there remains a group of Naturopaths who have digressed completely from the standardization implemented by the institutions and education of the professionalized, and thus may have a different relationship to the question regarding Foucault's anti-clinic. This group is described below.

2   "Come a Patient, Return a Doctor"

Looking at their histories, it is hard to pinpoint the precise event or point in time when the two schools of South Indian Naturopaths, professionalized and psycho-nutritionals, separated, since in the case of Kerala they have the same theoretical background. Psycho-nutritional education as a distinct concept only arose in the last twenty years in opposition to the trends of standardization and professionalization of practice.[10] In Kerala, all those interested in Naturopathy used to gather at the meetings of an organization called the All Kerala Nature Cure Federation (AKNCF).[11] In this organization, non-qualified people from different backgrounds with an interest in Naturopathy met regularly for conferences and talks. In the late 1990s, however, a small group drifted

---

10   A psycho-nutritional approach emerged in several institutions worldwide to describe the denial of psycho-pharmaceutical medication in the treatment of mental disorders. Instead, its followers recommend healing mental problems by means of adequate foods, which have the power to transform the chemicals in the brain (for more information see, for example, the Internet source Charis Holistic Center 2012). In the context of Kerala, however, it is an approach meant to describe not only remedies for mental disorders but for all kind of health problems. A connection between these streams was mentioned twice to me by psycho-nutritional practitioners. Most of the psycho-nutritionals stem from an academic circle of psychologists and other social scientist with an interest in diet, which might additionally explain the choice of naming. Although probably not all subsumed practitioners here would agree on the term psycho-nutritional to describe the approach, for the purpose of analysis, a distinction between professionals and non-professionals by the above term facilitates understanding.

11   There is hardly any written information in English on the All Kerala Nature Cure Federation, since their working language is exclusively Malayalam. The following information comes from current and former members of the federation collected through several interviews.

from the AKNCF and continued their practice at their homes and finally built their own hospitals.[12] This group cannot be characterized by its institutional organization. Rather, psycho-nutritionals form a very heterogeneous network, mainly in the geographical center and north of Kerala. While in the rest of India non-professionals constitute a marginalized group, in Kerala they are dominant due to their strong public presence in the media and their tendency to produce scandals.

The term psycho-nutritious education is derived from the academic work taking place at Kozhikode University in the field of psychology and related subjects. It describes a method of treatment consisting mainly of psychological approaches, nutritional treatment, and patient education on these topics (Kalayam 2008, Baby 2010, Baby 2004). Psycho-nutritionals are not a fixed group as such; it is more of an ideology, followed by people from more or less health-related sectors but with a clear preponderance of psychologists. Considering oneself part of this group does not necessarily mean actively treating patients, but rather refers to a supportive attitude towards the activities of the group members. Supporters are connected through several platforms, such as common events, media work, social groups on the Internet – such as Facebook, a group with 400 members in Kerala alone – and even community work in hospitals and ashrams.

The most prominent and charismatic figure of this group is Dr. Vadakkanchery, a social worker from Ernakulam. He and about fifty other activists form a loose network whose members organize conferences, camps, TV shows, and radio programs, and publish books and magazines. A series of twelve CDs featuring recordings of Dr. Vadakkanchery's speeches was released by the Nature Life Hospitals. These speeches are used in the hospitals for educating patients and can be purchased for around 200 rupees each. The psycho-nutritionals treat thousands of patients, though none of the healers have a medical degree in a strict sense.

Distinguishing the three characteristics of psycho-nutritionals – specifically, contesting globalization and "Western civilization," the principles of simplicity and transparency, and the underlying goal of empowerment – will enable psycho-nutritional education to be analyzed in more detail. These

---

12   Today the All Kerala Nature Cure Federation consists of a group of doctors with and without degrees, all practicing in a naturopathic hospital or consulting and treating patients privately. None of the non-degree AKNCF doctors operate their hospital without at least one BNYS doctor and they provide the infrastructure for internships and jobs for young BNYS scholars.

three characteristics, interlocking, fluid and co-determinant, represent the present ideological and material core of psycho-nutritional education.

The focus will be on Dr. Vadakkanchery as the mouthpiece of the psycho-nutritionals and the practices in Nature Life Hospitals, a chain of ten hospitals that he and his co-workers opened in India and Thailand in the late 1980s; a sixth clinic just recently opened in Kerala. The Nature Life group publishes a monthly magazine in Malayalam called *Sujeevitham*, which means "Good Life" in English. This magazine has recently boasted a circulation of 15,000 copies and is therefore widespread and very well-known in Kerala, according to an interview with Dr. Vadakkanchery in January 2011.

Contesting Globalization

Psycho-nutritionals promote not only Naturopathy as a treatment method but also what they see as a traditional Indian lifestyle, which they set in clear contrast to a so-called Western lifestyle. In general, they condemn the usage of all Western imports, referring to the most advertised and familiar "capitalist" products in Kerala such as Coca-Cola, denim jeans, and hygiene products, as well as cultural aspects such as styles of dress, architecture, behavior patterns, values, music, European languages (especially English), attitudes about personal liberty, sexuality and gender, and scientific and technological rationality. Psycho-nutritionals avoid drawing distinctions between the different religious groups present in Kerala. As Naturopathy is strongly regarded as a way of life, living according to its principles thus has moral implications. In order to express their rejection of "Western imperialism," psycho-nutritionals seek to promote and exemplify a life using only local products. Jacob Vadakkanchery, for instance, wears only one kind of apparel, an Indian-made white *kurta*. His definition of globalization is the "*meticulous scientific, psychological and anthropological planning which has been progressing for the last 50 years*" (Vadakkanchery CD 1, translation Indu P.). Globalization is seen as the result of imperialistic politics from the "West" with the goal of economically exploiting former colonized people. Modernity, conceptualized as a linear teleological line of "development" starting from Ancient Greece and intensifying in colonial and neocolonial times, is seen to be the key factor of globalization.

In general, psycho-nutritionals regard it as their mission to politically campaign against this form of neocolonialism in all its possible facets, but especially against "*Allopathy, which is the latest weapon of globalization*" (ibid). The antipathy directed at Allopathy and its treatments, medications, products and practitioners, is the main ingredient of Dr. Vadakkanchery's speeches. On the fourth CD of his series, he explains why this is so:

A doctor won't do anything to ensure the health of the patient since it will damage his job. The medical company bought him a car on the promise that he will prescribe 5000 tablets a day. Then how can he cure the patient? These doctors don't know anything about medicines. If they knew anything, at least they would remain healthy. Doctors are the people who suffer most from diseases (Vadakkanchery CD 4, translation Indu P.).

In Dr. Vadakkanchery's opinion, allopathic doctors are clearly aware of the fact that their medicine and treatments do not help the patient, but they dupe the patients intentionally for monetary interests:

A good doctor can identify the disease of the patient at first sight. By the time the doctor touches and speaks to that patient, he will be able to diagnose the disease properly. [...] Doctors are aware of the fact that most illnesses will be cured automatically without any special treatment. Here I say that all diseases will be cured in this way. [...] When the patient enters, the doctor glances at him. Then he realizes that the patient will be cured within two weeks. The doctor will conduct a few tests and say that you have to take medicines for a month. The patient is willing to take medicines since he doesn't know that the disease doesn't require any special treatment. So he takes the medicines. Whatever may be the treatment, he gets cured before two weeks. The patient will think that the doctor is so efficient that he got cured quickly. The doctor who is able to instill this belief in a patient will succeed (Vadakkanchery CD 3, translation Indu P.).

This quote shows the extent to which psycho-nutritionals believe in the malpractice, corruption and dishonest intentions of allopathic doctors. According to Dr. John Baby, another follower of the psycho-nutritional philosophy with a PhD in psychology, medical companies spend money to influence the media in order to prevent them from spreading the message of the non-medical naturopathic treatments. Dr. Baby, Dr. Vadakkanchery and other psycho-nutritionals promote the opinion that allopathic medical companies are actively to blame for withholding information about the effectiveness of Naturopathy because it would create strong competition in the market. If allopathic doctors had a real interest in the health of their patients, they would therefore turn towards Naturopathy. Three examples will illustrate the ideology followed by psycho-nutritionals, two of them from the monthly magazine *Sujeevitham* and the other from the counter-campaign to Pulse Polio, a vaccination campaign run by the Indian Ministry of Health.

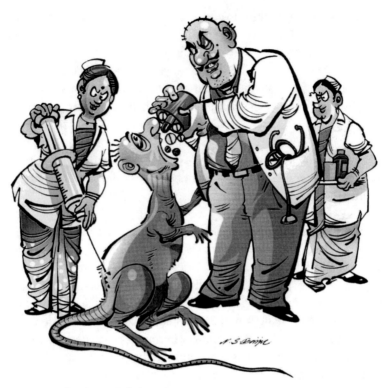

FIGURE 4   *"India, the Land of Pharma Drug Experiments"*

First, a visual critique of allopathic practices adorned the cover of the magazine *Sujeevitham* (translated as "Good Life") in October 2008 (Figure 4).

The patient is illustrated as a helpless laboratory rat, surrounded by sinister
allopathic practitioners who are forcing invasive and random medication into
both sides of the patient. The caricaturist paints the doctor in front as a sadis-
tic-looking man, dressed in Western clothes with a tie and a shirt under his
white coat. The nurses or female assistants in the back are Indians represented
through the bindi spots on their foreheads and the saris they are wearing.
However, the white coat and the white cap conceal this Indianness at first
glance and therefore they could be perceived as collaborators, masking their
true identity. One of the nurses is injecting an unknown liquid into the back of
the patient, while the other, smiling maliciously, fetches more medication. The
patient in the very front has a hairy chimeric appearance. He obviously has
very limited capacity to act due to his excessively short and atrophied arms,
which make it impossible for him to struggle. The title of the drawing, "India,
the Land of Pharma Drug Experiments," enforces the impression that the

Allopaths depicted here act arbitrarily and only for their own advantage. The message is clear: Allopathy abuses the Indian population by making them the key market for medical experiments.

The second example is a counter-campaign run by the psycho-nutritionals against polio vaccination in Kerala. Since vaccination was already the cause of much tension during colonialism, this contemporary struggle has a major historical precedent. During my fieldwork in 2010 in Kerala, the Ministry of Health in India initiated a campaign against polio and placed information booths in the bus stations of middle-sized towns, where young associates with yellow caps undertook awareness-raising in the form of disseminating flyers, conducting counseling interviews and even providing on-site oral vaccinations. This was a follow-up campaign to a similar "Pulse Polio" initiative in 1994. Immediately, a small group of psycho-nutritionals published a counterattack flyer entitled "Discard Pulse Polio." On this flyer, they cited studies by several medical experts within and outside India, both allopathic and naturopathic, who argued against the effectiveness of the oral polio vaccination. In addition, psycho-nutritional researchers published statistics about patients proving the failure of the campaign in the years since 1994 and highlighting the risk of VAPP (Vaccine-Associated Paralytic Poliomyelitis), a possible side effect of polio vaccination. According to the flyer, the reason the government gives oral vaccinations for free, although they are fairly aware of the dangerous and even deadly side effects, is that the pharmaceutical companies want to conduct trials with a large proportion of the population without paying fees to the probands. In this view, pharmaceutical companies are the drivers behind the acts of the government but they are still conspiring with each other in order to mutually maximize their profit.

As a third example I would like to refer once again to *Sujeevitham*, the magazine of the Nature Life Hospital group. In October 2009, right after the dramatic death of Michael Jackson, *Sujeevitham* published the cover depicted in Figure 5. On this cover Michael Jackson is depicted in before-and-after views. On the right-hand side, his skin color is significantly lighter than in the photograph on the left. The most peculiar thing about the two photographs is the significant change in his nose: Even if Jackson's nose in the picture on the left is different from what appears in his childhood pictures, it still looks somehow normal and healthy, while in the other picture such drastic changes have been made that it does not even seem to belong to his face. Jackson's eyes look big and empty and are framed by dark sockets. The issue of the magazine is titled *"How Biomedicine Killed Michael Jackson."* As the name suggests, the cover story – written by Dr. Vadakkanchery – traces in detail the steps that led to Michael Jackson's poisoning and finally to his death. As Dr.

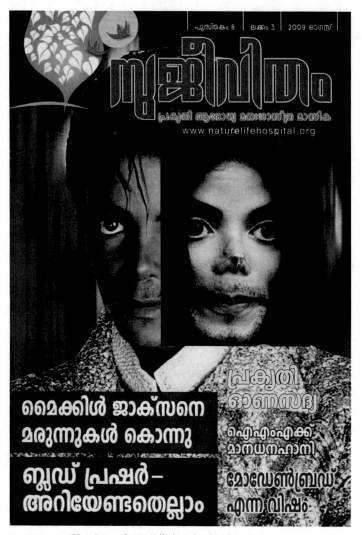

FIGURE 5   *"How Biomedicine Killed Michael Jackson"*

Vadakkanchery explains, in 1984 *"Jackson's face was not ugly, till then it was cute and masculine at the same time"* (Vadakkanchery 2009: 7-8, translation by Indu P.). Jackson suffered burns and injuries related to a smoke bomb explosion on stage and subsequently began to take strong painkillers to relieve his pain, which ultimately resulted in addiction. In Dr. Vadakkanchery's perspective, allopathic medical practitioners' actions made him an addict. He began to take an increasing number of tablets: *"Tablets for acidity, antibiotics, sleeping pills, tablets to boost energy levels, tablets for proper digestion, tablets to reduce ten-sion, tablets to recover from depression, all these made Jackson 'Medicine' Jackson"* (ibid). He is not entirely sure if it was the immense influence of allopathic doc-tors that induced 'Medicine' Jackson to undergo all of his 13 plastic surgeries or if it was the confusion caused by his strong medications. In any case, it was the allopathic doctors who *"accumulated a great fortune by subjecting him to 13 plastic surgeries. The surgeries made his face uglier and opened Jackson's wallet for the next one"* (ibid). Dr. Vadakkanchery summarizes the unfortunate case of 'Medicine' Jackson as follows:

> After the treatment for burns, Jackson was dragged into the vortex of con-troversies. The allopathic medicines he used for the treatment led to the deviance in his behavior and in the end resulted in his premature death. Michael Jackson is an unfortunate example of how allopathic medicine makes a man go astray, how it makes him commit crimes and how it tor-tures him by making him a patient for the rest of his life. When we check the medicines prescribed for Jackson, we can understand that he is not the only catastrophe and it is a disaster that falls upon all those who take allopathic medicines (ibid).

Psycho-nutritionals took the opportunity presented by Michael Jackson's death and the subsequent discussion on the causes of his demise in order to propagate their dismissive opinion about any kind of allopathic treatment. Michael Jackson, who had black skin by birth but was *"transformed"* into a white person by allopathic doctors, therefore fulfills the role of shunning the *"local"* (in other words, his "origin" as symbolized through the color of his skin) with the help of allopathic practitioners, and through this he became ugly and poor.

Psycho-nutritionals use means that attract public attention. Through the strategic adoption of media strategies, be it flyers, their own newspaper or even TV programs, they pick up current topics and operationalize them for the promotion of their own practice. Although their main target is clearly allo-pathic practices, they also use these outlets to charge other professionalized medical systems such as Ayurveda or Siddha with commercialization.

As depicted in Table 2, in 2006 Bode[13] delineated the simplified, dichoto-mous view of allopathic medicine in comparison to "traditional" knowledge. Although it might seem like a contradiction, since Bode referred in his article to the creation of an Indian identity by production of Ayurveda and Unani

---

13   Bode 2006: 232

TABLE 2   *"Stereotypes of Western and Indian Medicine"*

Type of Medical System	Stereotypes			
Western	Commerce, greed	Industry	Exploitation	Aggression
Indian	Altruism, compassion	Nature	Sustenance	Gentleness

pharmaceuticals, Table 2 clearly summarizes the way psycho-nutritionals differentiate their own practice from all other practices (including professionalized Naturopathy). Standardization and professionalization mean that medical systems such as Ayurveda, Unani and Siddha rank among Western systems of medicine for them. Naturopathy, on the other hand, is seen as authentic, natural, and wholesome, and therefore as the only legitimate form of treatment, linked at its essence to Indian culture through the influence of Mahatma Gandhi and other Indian pioneers.

Simplicity and Transparency

A distinctive characteristic of psycho-nutritionals is that they regard their practice as a social vocation, rather than a profession. The goal of these Naturopaths is to dedicate themselves to promoting general welfare. However, the costs of the psycho-nutritional cure vary and depend on the duration of the treatment or event and on the location of treatment; organizers never tire of assuring patients or participants that their fees only cover costs. In their opinion, BNYS doctors generally do not act in this way; instead, they are money- and career-orientated, and psycho-nutritionals want to differentiate themselves from that ideology.

Education within psycho-nutritional circles is quite heterogeneous in contrast to that of the BNYS doctor: Most psycho-nutritionals are autodidacts who have acquired knowledge without any formal education. New followers are recruited at events and in hospitals, in most cases former patients – some of them already labeled as incurable – who were healed and convinced by Naturopathy. Since 2010, Dr. Vadakkanchery and his associates have been running their own education center in his hospital in Ernakulam in order to recruit assistants for his treatments. The duration of the course is between two months and two years, and afterwards the apprentices are sent to one of his hospitals. This form of education mainly focuses on substance-related treatments. Other co-workers in the hospital have a DNYT degree or receive a similar short-term education program in Naturopathy. There is even one BNYS degree-holder, as an employee of a Nature Life Hospital once confessed with shame. However, in the opinion of psycho-nutritionals, this medical degree proves to be more of a disadvantage for the BNYS scholar, since the logic of medical hierarchy is already instilled in this doctor and has to be unlearned.

In order to understand psycho-nutritional ideology, psycho-nutritionals consistently emphasize that long-term education is not necessary. On the contrary, it is the nature of the psycho-nutritional cure that it can be understood quickly and easily by everyone. The transmission of knowledge is therefore not limited to an elite that has the intellectual and financial capacity to spend five years or longer in advanced education. Transparency is maintained through the simplicity of the education, and is evident in the treatments given to the patients.

Dr. John Baby places a strong emphasis on the fact that people in the "modern world" have estranged themselves from nature by turning away from the five elements. In his view, simplicity means living according to the guidelines of the essential elements: a supply of oxygen, the consumption of cold water, or walking barefoot on the earth.

In order to make this clear, an animal model is pointed out by naturopathic practitioners quite often. In several of my interviews, Naturopaths explained human similarities to vegetarian animals as proof of nature's intention for human nutrition. Others observed animals (such as wild dogs or cows) in order to learn from their behavior. Public talks and written publications by Naturopaths are full of comparisons with the animal world, where non-human creatures are offered as the finest example of "good living." The forest is thereby an imaginary place, where natural and "good living" takes place.

This is Dr. Baby's idea of simplicity, taking in the minimum means that are available for everybody. All patients in psycho-nutritional camps or hospitals therefore receive the same food, which is easily available locally. Patients receive only a minimum of additional treatments, since those are difficult to use at home. Psycho-nutritionals explain treatments, their efficacy and purpose in fine detail to the patient with the explicit expectation that the patient must understand his or her own body and its diseases in order to apply that knowledge later at home. Thus, a return visit to a naturopathic hospital would theoretically become unnecessary. This is indeed the most striking factor of the psycho-nutritional approach: Their method of treatment is intended to be self-sufficient. As soon as patients have learned the "true" way of living, they are able to implement and even to teach that knowledge for the rest of their lives. This practice is implemented in the slogan "come a patient, return a doctor." The naturopathic claim to abolish disease and hospitals long-term through medical education, prevention, and clarification is unique among the medical systems existing in South India.

"Empowerment"

Contesting globalization and the motif of simplicity both underlie a higher goal: Empowerment of the people. In Dr. Vadakkanchery's words: "*I am against the government and the system and the power, I want people to take their own power so I want to weaken that system. A self-governing system, like Gandhi said, self-ruled.*" By rejecting all Western imports and implementing simplicity, the everyday simplicity that everybody can achieve, the agency of the people is supposed to be strengthened. Psycho-nutritionals place the political signifi-cance of Naturopathy in the context of the Gandhian freedom movement and highlight its historical struggle against untouchability and alcoholism and for the empowerment of women and lower classes.

This egalitarian approach is expressed in practice, for example, through sev-eral intermarriages (primarily Hindu-Christian) by psycho-nutritionals, an undertaking that in conservative Kerala has very often resulted in sanctions by their families. However, those involved in intermarriages legitimize them not by the motif of the new middle-class concept of love, but rather by a common interest in Naturopathy and its ideology.

Following Naturopathy treatments and adapting to its way of life enables "ordinary people" to free their minds to reach a mental and physical state where they are able to regard globalization in realistic terms – in other words, to see it for what it truly is. Psycho-nutritionals also distrust established insti-tutions, political and economic power structures and media. These power structures oppress Naturopathy practices that are based on self-rule, self-reli-ability, self-governing and self-contained ideas. Naturopathy offers a direct challenge to Allopathy, with the stated intention to "free" people from the pres-sure to buy and consume.

With this in mind, the before-mentioned three examples can be analyzed in a more explicit way. In the case of the patient-turned-lab rat, his helplessness and lack of agency is symbolized by the fact that his arms are atrophied. A laboratory rat is normally not aware of the disease it is infected with, and is therefore not able to take a critical look at the doctor's actions. It is thus completely at the mercy of the allopathic doctors and unable to make free and informed decisions. In the example of the Indian government's Pulse Polio vaccination campaign, the psycho-nutritionals are highly skeptical about campaign workers showing up at bus stations and "experimenting" on people by giving them on-site vaccinations. Since the probands are not aware that they are – once again – being turned into laboratory rats, they have no influence on their destiny. In the case of 'Medicine' Jackson, it was not directly him and his will that made him undergo countless operations. It was the confusion he was trapped in after taking all the allopathic medicines and the manipulative power that cash-hungry allopathic doctors wielded over him. The laboratory rat, the involuntarily-vaccinated probands and 'Medicine' Jackson were all turned into passive, unempowered objects through the imperialistic methods of allopathic medicine.

Looking at the presentations of psycho-nutritionals, it becomes evident that they consider the body not to be a docile, passive entity but rather a self-governing body. In this view, biopower should not lie within the state or its institutions but within its population. With these assumptions as its foundation, Naturopathy becomes a complete and radical alternative to all other medical systems present in India. In theory, according to Alter (2004), remedial health care would eventually become obsolete with a continuing dissemination of naturopathic knowledge. However, the caveat to this statement is that Naturopathy is not at all a homogenous practice. In the case of professionalized Naturopathy, empowerment and the strengthening of the self-governing body is not volitional and not even promoted. Instead, professionalized Naturopathy aims to restrict the ownership of knowledge to specialists, a position that fits Foucault's description of biopower as handled by the modern nation state.

In its ideal state, psycho-nutritionals' practice does not depend on capitalism, production and nationalism. This group intends to replicate itself through the production of more and more doctors until a large network is established that can perpetuate itself through its increasing number of participants. However, since psycho-nutritionals are realistic enough to recognize the fact that the literal "natural state" is still far off, in the meantime they concentrate on disseminating their messages.

3 Sudden Crisis of Naturopathy: Registration Politics

Until their split in the AKNCF, professional Naturopaths and psycho-nutritionals had coexisted for the last two decades in Kerala. Only in the beginning of the 2000s did this relatively peaceful coexistence turn divisive when government institutions introduced legal registration for professional naturopathic practitioners. This move had significant implications for psycho-nutritionals since the perceived legitimacy of a medical system, as well as governmental and public acceptance, is often linked to its legal status.

After finishing their education at an appropriate institution, AYUSH practitioners register to practice their brand of medicine. An exception is Naturopathy in Kerala. In Kerala, naturopathic legal registration for BNYS doctors was only introduced in November 2010. The official explanation for this is the lack of colleges in Kerala; in surrounding states like Tamil Nadu and Maharashtra, legal registration was introduced two decades ago. BNYS graduates register at the state offices right after attaining their degree and receive an A-class registration.[14] A Naturopath trained for five years outside of Kerala was therefore only legally equated with the category of medical "lay practitioner," which includes such diverse workers as astrologers, priests, or a housewife with an interest in collecting herbs for her neighbors.

It was the following incident that triggered discussion on legal acceptance in Kerala: At the end of the 1990s a young woman named Parvati[15] discovered a tumor in her breast. Parvati at that time was part of a circle of acquaintances following psycho-nutritional ideology and was a regular visitor and attendee of psycho-nutritional health camps. She first turned to homeopathic treatment for two or three years until she finally decided to change her personal relationship with the psycho-nutritionals into a doctor-patient relationship. She turned to one of her fellow psycho-nutritionals, Aneesh, and asked for his help. For many years, Parvati had had a close relationship with him and his family. Aneesh's wife, having always been very critical towards Naturopathy, wanted to send her to a hospital immediately to get a proper allopathic diagnosis for the developing tumor, since she doubted that the curing power of naturopathic treatment would be enough for a tumor in this advanced stage. Parvati and Aneesh, however, decided together that she would undergo naturopathic treatment. Aneesh did not believe in the possibility of cancer; according to him Parvati was simply suffering from a scab. Parvati attended a 7-day health camp, followed by a 40-day fruitarian diet and finally received treatment in a naturopathic hospital. According to critical observers she did not follow naturopathic principles in a proper way and ate cooked food and even fish in between the diets. Parvati's tumor did not disappear. She was disappointed and began to blame Aneesh's naturopathic treatment publicly for the failure. Since she had a background with the Communist Party, the case took

---

14 Ayurveda was the first medical system to register its practitioners in order to delineate professionals from quacks. They used two different forms of registration: An A-class registration for BAMS, meaning college-educated practitioners, and a B-class registration for accepted *vaidyas*. The admittance for these non-College-trained ayurvedic practitioners varied over different periods of time but shows a strong trend towards becoming stricter (Kaiser 1992).

15 Since this incident had very negative effects on the careers and personal lives of all those involved and their families, the names of the people concerned have been changed.

on political overtones in Kerala. Newspapers such as the Madhyamam approached Parvati for interviews and wrote articles about the incident. These articles featured lurid headlines like *"Did he treat her as a guinea pig hiding her disease?"* In press conferences and on TV, Parvati accused Aneesh of having experimented with her health since he did not have any proper experience in the treatment of cancer (Jannabhumi Daily, May 2005). Aneesh, however, suspected her of not following naturopathic principles in a way that would have led to her cure. Nevertheless, his reputation was damaged to such a degree that he was suspended from his workplace, where he held a high-ranking position, until a Research Committee could clarify the circumstances of Parvati's failure of treatment and Aneesh's role in it. The case became more delicate when Parvati finally died in 2005 after a long series of chemotherapies.

The case was torn to pieces by the media inside and outside of Kerala. People on the street expressed a variety of opinions. Aneesh's colleagues and supporters started demonstrations and hunger strikes in front of his workplace in order to protest against the suspension. The case even found its way into the High Court of Kerala but was dismissed. It took almost five more years until the reproaches were revoked and Aneesh was declared not guilty in the death of Parvati. In the meantime, professional Naturopaths began to defend themselves against accusations that were brought against Naturopathy as an entire system. They started arguing for an institutionalized classification of Naturopaths. This brought up the question of practitioners' registration in Kerala and finally led to its implementation. Since the introduction of legal acceptance in November 2010 by AYUSH, the two groups of naturopathic practitioners have been differentiated on an institutionalized basis: Professionals were legalized by the government to treat patients. Since psycho-nutritionals do not have the official BNYS degree, they were refused registration.

However, not long after this in the spring of 2011, driven by private institutions qualifying students with DNYT or other degrees in Naturopathy, the government of Kerala proposed a B-class registration. This brought up the memory of Parvati's death in the context of psycho-nutritional cures and, initiated by INYGMA, 250 BNYS students from the neighboring states of Tamil Nadu and Maharashtra gathered in front of the city hall in the capital of Kerala, Thiruvananthapuram, to protest against the introduction of another form of registration and therefore legal acceptance of any degree other than the state-regulated BNYS. Rumors about the corruption of government institutes by different members of the psycho-nutritional movement were widespread. Figure 6 depicts one example from the newspaper *Malayalam Manorama*:[16]

---

16   Malayalam Manorama 2011, February 4th.

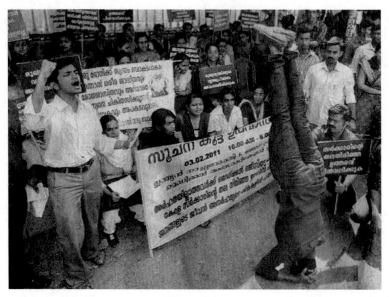

FIGURE 6   *Students of BNYS protesting*

The students were pretty worked up, conducting Yoga *asanas* in protest and holding protest signs announcing a group hunger strike.[17] They were protesting against the corruptibility of the government of Kerala, assuming that the Prime Minister – by virtue of the fact that he was once on the cover of *Sujeevitham* and has the reputation of being very close to Jacob Vadakkanchery – takes money from the psycho-nutritionals in order to give them legal registration outside of the BNYS A-class registration. Moreover, BNYS students were acting on the assumption that the DYNT course, due to be opened for B-class registration by the government, could be attained in only three days. Participants of the strike considered a psycho-nutritional Naturopathy to be unwelcome competition, since psycho-nutritionals also call themselves Naturopaths. College-educated Naturopaths, however, do not want to be associated with them. They feel that their good reputation and long education is threatened by what they call non-qualified quacks. One of the participants reproached Dr. Vadakkanchery for not having adequate knowledge in anatomy and phys-

---

17   Some translations from the signs (Indu P.): "*Withdraw the decision to provide medical registration to those who do not deserve it.*" "*People's lives are not a toy to be played with by undeserving fellows.*" "*Put an end to ministers' pseudo-attempts to please.*" "*Government orders are being implemented. Fake courses are multiplying. Knowledge is shrinking. People are getting screwed.*"

iology. From this perspective, Dr. Vadakkanchery's lack of knowledge has caused people to die in the past and – if nobody stops him – they will continue to die in the future. Another active member of INYGMA summarized their approach as follows:

> It is very necessary that we have professional knowledge, medical knowl-
> edge, otherwise we don't know what is happening in the body. If we don't
> know physiology and biochemistry, then how can we treat the patient?
> With the BNYS they receive proper knowledge and at the same time
> proper application. Without a degree and registration they are just
> blindly applying treatment without knowing what is happening in the
> body. So this is the problem and we are fighting against these quacks.

This strike was the first public event organized by INYGMA for BNYS students and practitioners with the intention of delineating themselves from non-qual-ified practitioners. The outcome of the strike was that the government took back their proposal with the promise to review it, and so far BNYS doctors are the only ones to benefit from legal registration.

Psycho-nutritional cures are not entirely legal, but fall into a gray zone, because it is hard to criminalize people recommending that you eat raw food and avoid chemicals. Jacob Vadakkanchery himself maintains a low profile about the introduction of B-class registration and the strikes by the BNYS stu-dents in Thiruvananthapuram. He denies that he is indeed the initiator of the suggested B-class registration. On the contrary, on being asked about the issue of registration, Dr. Vadakkanchery says:

> I am not worried about registration, we don't want the government noti-
> fication or registration; I am not going to get it, I don't want the license of
> the government. I am not a slave of the government. There's no need for
> that. I will not support the government and the system and the power.

According to Dr. Vadakkanchery, there is no need for psycho-nutritionals to be involved in the whole discussion on registration since it has no effect on their practice but would in fact restrict it further by forcing them to comply with government regulations. Dr. Vadakkanchery's approach is more idealistic than that: He wants people to learn and understand their body and treatment in order to be self-ruled in the healing process. He does not want them to be ruled by physicians, whether allopathic or BNYS.

4   Conclusion

This chapter has illustrated two very different approaches to Naturopathy in Kerala. Although both streams rely on similar ideas of health and disease and use the same books as the foundation for their ideology and treatments, their representation of Naturopathy differs. Nowadays, professional Naturopathy is strongly based on the global flows of allopathic principles such as anatomy and physiology, but only uses naturopathic treatments to heal ailments. They have established a medical norm that is congruent with the prevalent medical norm – Allopathy – and therefore fits into Foucault's analysis of the clinic. By "scientificating," institutionalizing and professionalizing Naturopathy, BNYS doctors have created a medical system that is based on the transmission of special knowledge, which cannot be accessed and learned by everybody but only by an elite who can afford the education. In this context there is a strong connection between expert medical knowledge and the power that profes-sional naturopathic practitioners gain over the bodies and healing processes of their patients. They are thereby able to commercialize the act of healing as a service and to compete with other medical systems on the market such as Ayurveda, Allopathy or Unani. Professionals aim to integrate themselves into a new technological medical world by taking some of the old weapons and shap-ing them for the modern environment.

The approach of the psycho-nutritionals differs greatly. In contrast to the professionals, their agenda can be understood in a framework of political activ-ism: In the tradition of Gandhi, the application of the genuine Indian medical system of Naturopathy should provide self-determination in post-colonial India. The transmission of agency from the doctor to the patient as well as psycho-nutritionals' construction of a different kind of normativity, namely life in tune with nature as a higher goal, are main characteristics of what Alter (2004) termed the anti-clinic. Naturopathy for psycho-nutritionals is more than a medical system: It is intended to change society. In order to maintain authenticity, it is imperative that any kind of commercialization, whether medication or services, is denied. The motives of anybody who makes money from Naturopathy are generally contested. The differences between both streams become most obvious and visible in the context of legal registration, an ongoing conflict in Kerala.

CHAPTER 4

Naturopathic Spaces: On Nutrition, Substances and Psychological Integration

Research in hospitals or about hospitals did not begin to attract much attention by social scientists until the 1970s, when Michel Foucault presented his influential historical analysis on the development of allopathic hospitals in Europe and their function as exclusive and excluding institutional spaces (Foucault 1973). In *The Birth of the Clinic*, Foucault critiqued earlier ethnographic work that analyzed hospitals as bounded entities or islands, cut off from the rest of the world where "normal life" takes place (e.g., Goffman 1961, Coser 1962). The latter approach correlated at that time with ethnographies about villages or small communities, but in Foucault's view failed to account for the larger picture in which healing practices take place, which are shaped by power asymmetries and biopolitics. Influenced by these critiques, more recent ethnographic work conceptualizes hospitals as entities that reflect and mirror existing social structures – in other words, the notion of the hospital as a microcosm of society or the "hospital as culturally-embedded" (Zaman 2005, van der Geest and Finkler 2004). In the relevant literature on the study of hospitals, these two positions operate on two ends of a continuum that encompasses a range of perspectives regarding the nature of the relationship between social structures and the hospital, and the permeability of the boundaries between the two (Street and Coleman 2012).

The past several decades have seen hospital ethnographies emerge as a trend in modern anthropology. This trend was preceded by the identification and articulation of Allopathy as just one cultural system alongside other local medical systems (see, for example, Gaines and Hahn 1985, Good 1995, Hahn and Kleinman 1983, Lindenbaum and Lock 1993, Rhodes 1990). Anthropologists have examined the flexible accommodations made by hospital staff and patients to resource constraints in non-Western countries, such as Brown's (2012) examination of the mobilization of the extended family in Kenya, Livingston's (2012) research in a Botswana oncology ward, Street's (2011, 2014) study on fragile hospital infrastructures in Papua New Guinea, and Zaman's (2004, 2005) research in Bangladesh on the frustration resulting from a lack of resources. Other investigations pertain to the dependence of hospitals on the state, such as Sullivan's (2012) study of hospital financing in Tanzania, Gibson's (2004) writings on the medical gaze and state surveillance in South African

© KONINKLIJKE BRILL NV, LEIDEN, 2016 | DOI 10.1163/9789004325104_007

hospitals, Addlakha's (2008) description of a clash between government-paid health workers and patients with mental illness in North India, and Nichter's (1986) investigation of primary health care centers, likewise in India.

In all of these approaches, the hospital is conceptualized as the ultimate center where medical knowledge (typically allopathic) is produced and reproduced, and where practices are implemented. As van der Geest and Finkler (2004) suggest, there exists not just one allopathic system, model or school but rather a diversity of allopathic theories and practices, appropriated through global flows in different contexts. Scholars such as Andersen (2004) with his study on differential treatment in a hospital in Ghana, and Mol (2002) with her research on atherosclerosis diagnosis and treatment in a Dutch hospital, show that even within the biomedical paradigm, the notion of the body and healing can differ enormously.

Despite the growing literature on allopathic hospitals in non-Western settings, only a few researchers have engaged with translations between medical systems. Langwick's (2008) study on the concurrence of "traditional" and "modern" medicine in Tanzania, Quack and Chopra's (2011) writing on psychiatry and Ayurveda, and Lang's (2014) research with Muslim healers and psychology (the latter three authors all in India) are of mention here. Surprisingly, little research has been conducted in "pure" non-allopathic hospitals. Two of the rare exceptions are Langford's (2002) research on ayurvedic hospitals in India and Farquhar's (1994) work on Chinese medicine in the 1980s.

In order to define the qualities of naturopathic practices, I refer to the work of Agic (2012), who conducted his research on the use of mechanical hearts in Sweden, and Street and Coleman (2012), authors of the introduction to *Hospital Heterotopias: Ethnographies of Biomedical and Non-Biomedical Spaces*. All three authors refer to the concept of Foucault's heterotopia (1986). According to the latter, an archetypal heterotopia is an anomaly of everyday life, or a parallel, non-hegemonic space that occurs within an institution in society. The hospital constitutes such a parallel space of otherness, removing from society those whose sickness or behavior falls outside the hegemonic norm. A heterotopia follows rules of discipline and surveillance, just like other institutions examined by Foucault. Agic (2012) talked about his ward as the "other space," arguing that it possessed its own body of rules, social standards and rites of purification. Street and Coleman (2012) specified and expanded this concept; according to them, hospitals consist of "*multiple internal and external spaces whose relationships change over time with shifting configurations of actors*" (Street and Coleman 2012:9). Therefore, hospital spaces are processual, transformative, permeable, innovative, multilayered, and constantly incomplete.

I interpret "naturopathic spaces" in this ambiguous and contradictory way. Not only is the naturopathic space a "village" with its own set of rules and rites, but it is also a microcosm of society as well as a globalized, permeable entity.

While in many parts of the world non-allopathic therapy might not be institutionalized to the same degree as allopathic, Naturopathy has a similarly specialized division of labor and is localized to comparatively long-existing sites in India. Furthermore, Indian naturopathic practitioners distinguish between outpatient and hospital treatment, as their allopathic colleagues do. Therefore, physical demarcation is crucial in both allopathic and naturopathic contexts. A hospital is characterized either as a detached building or as a campus with visible boundaries separating it from "the rest of the world." In contrast to public space, it has specific entrance rules and is only open for specific groups of people with similar dispositions.

I define "naturopathic spaces" indeed within the physical bounds of the hospital. This is the heart of naturopathic practice, where increasing numbers of patients reflect the success of media and Internet work, and it is the hub that finances other naturopathic activities. It is also the place where certain (but not all) characteristics of society are reflected – social stratification is one example that will be addressed in subsequent chapters. A naturopathic hospital has permeable passages to all spaces where naturopathic theories and practices are interpreted, hybridized and implemented: advisory centers, health camps, social gatherings, political movements or groups, walk-in clinics or even conferences, where new knowledge is generated. The intriguing characteristic of Naturopathy is its entanglement with social, political and environmental movements with common ideologies, actors and masterminds. Therefore it can only be fluid, processual and incomplete. In this book, I consider Naturopathy framed in its historical and socio-cultural development. Naturopathy consists of circumscribable spaces that possess their own deviant rules of power, order, stability and continuity, which will be described throughout the remaining chapters.

This chapter is about two different naturopathic spaces. The first is the Gandhiji Naturopathy Hospital (GNH), close to Thrissur, run by Mr. Kalyan Ulpalakshan and his wife, a college-trained Naturopath with a BNYS degree. It can thus be regarded as an example of a professional hospital practice. Less than four hours away by bus is the second site of investigation, the Nature Life Hospital (NLH) in Kozhikode, a hospital run by the psycho-nutritionals Dr. Vadakkanchery and his wife. An examination of the daily routine in these hospitals reveals their implicit goals and orientation. By means of an analytical tripartition of naturopathic treatments into psychological integration, nutritional therapy and substance-related treatments, I will further examine and compare the practices in the two hospitals.

1   Gandhiji Naturopathy Hospital, Thrissur

The Gandhiji Naturopathy Hospital (GNH) is located on the outskirts of Thrissur, four kilometers away from the main station, on a small side road. The building itself is unpretentious, a green block containing four floors and a small courtyard at the back. The last renovation was some time ago, since the paint is peeling off the walls, some toilets lack seats, and other aspects of the building are in disrepair – for example, my bathroom window was broken, providing open access for the whole diversity of insects in Kerala. There are no buckets in the toilet, which is very uncommon for Indian bathrooms and it took me quite a while to figure out that patients are supposed to bring their own plates, glasses, buckets and sheets. Similarly, everything in this hospital is kept at a very basic level; comfort is not a top priority here. Rooms are fitted with meager furnishings: two beds in each room, narrow, short and uncomfortable mattresses and worn leather pillows await the patients. The only shelf in the room is lined with newspaper and a layer of dust. Eventually the reason for this neglect becomes clear: There are too many sick people for the available facilities, and Kalayan Ulpalakshan and his team are favored for their treatment. There is simply not enough money to take care of all of the necessary renovations and the maintenance of the building.

The GNH specializes in renal treatments, a focus that becomes more clear when one looks at its history: Professor Ulpalakshan, a former college teacher, suffered from renal failure and started curing himself successfully by using only naturopathic remedies. Subsequently, at the beginning of the 1980s, he decided to promote this treatment on a wider scale and founded an ashramlike hospital on the other side of the main street from the GNH. Here sick people gathered to live together and cure their diseases. Some years later the location was shifted and the current building was erected in 1999. There are three doctors in the current site: Kalyan Ulpalakshan, the son of the founder, his wife Dr. Jyotsana KS,[1] a BNYS degree-holder, and an alternating assistant, also from a BNYS college in his or her practical year. Kalyan Ulpalakshan learned about Naturopathy and the treatment of renal failure both from his father and from

---

1   In the subsequent sections, I will refer to all psycho-nutritionals and professionals as "Dr." who introduced themselves as such to myself and others. It is a reference to their profession as physician rather than the title of having a PhD or medical degree.

decades of experience. He does not have a health-related college or university degree and therefore does not officially wear the title of professor or doctor but is sometimes assigned both by patients and other practitioners because of his healing abilities, similar to the title previously awarded to his father. He has a soothing, wise manner when relating to the patients and running the hospital, leaving no doubt about his authority and expertise. The GNH is a typical example of the changes that are happening within Naturopathy: due to increasing professionalization, so-called autodidacts who had a treatment center before the trend commenced are now bringing young BNYS-educated doctors on board to lend an air of legitimacy to their practices.

The hospital is funded by a trust, a set-up that is quite common for Naturopathy hospitals (Alter 2004). The trust is fueled by unknown sources – or at least sources that are kept confidential by the management. This is part of a larger pattern: In general, many issues are kept confidential in this hospital from both patients as well as from myself when I was there as a researcher. Indeed, it was the only hospital during my research where inspection of case histories and file sheets was forbidden and many treatments remained unexplained.

In the lower floor, there are eight rooms for patients and one for the BNYS assistant, who resides in the hospital. An office for consultations with doctors is located at the very front. This room is fully monopolized by the doctors and is not supposed to be used by visitors, with the exception of invited patients, bystanders or guests who are there for consultation or examination. As van der Geest and Finkler (2004) suggest, this reticence in allowing outsiders or observers into an authorized space is a typical feature of allopathic hospitals. This also explains why I was never allowed to take part in any consultations or examinations in this room, except for my interviews with the doctors themselves.

At the back of the ground floor, there is a kitchen and separate mudpack room. Three women at a time manage the kitchen and prepare food for the patients and bystanders. In the entrance hall, there are two lines of chairs, used by the patients to chat with each other or to read newspapers. Outside, in front of the hospital, there is a bench that is used in a similar way but mainly by Tamil-speaking patients. On the first floor, there are another eleven rooms and a corridor large enough to accommodate more patients. They sleep on discarded or provisional beds in the midst of the daily hustle and bustle of the hospital. During my research, there were two or three patients at a time taking advantage of that option. There are sixteen rooms on the third floor and a narrow corridor with a TV in the middle, which attracts patients from all floors every evening for the daily soap operas playing on the Malayalam channel.

Some patients bring their own televisions for their rooms because there is not enough space for everybody in the corridor. On the fourth floor, there are only six rooms and a larger area dedicated for Yoga *asanas*. Due to a lack of interest on the part of patients and a scarcity of time to teach it, Yoga *asanas* take place very rarely. The intern at that time noted that Yoga would be only conducted for patients with mental ailments and at the time they did not have any, or at least none that were willing to do Yoga *asanas*. On the same floor there is a room for gymnastics with a single huge gym machine, but I have only seen it in use to hang wet laundry for drying. There are small attempts to ameliorate the condition of the building, such as renovating single rooms, but due to a constant shortage of money, progress on this front has been slow. Two rooms are fitted with air-conditioning and are therefore subject to a higher rent of 400 rupees rather than the usual tariff of 250 rupees per day. According to Dr. Jyotsana KS, this would never be sufficient without the aid of the trust, which provides the financial basis to finance the food.

Books written by Kalyan Ulpalakshan about Naturopathy can be found all over the hospital, as well as a quarterly magazine with articles on health and disease, published by the GNH in Malayalam. Every morning a variety of newspapers is delivered and shared by the patients on the bench in front of the hospital. Outside the gate, a clever businessman has opened a small tea and idli stall in order to feed the bystanders or renegade patients in the early mornings.

The GNH employs a number of helpers, ranging from administrative staff to kitchen staff and cleaners, in addition to about six women from the neighborhood who do the massages. All employees except the cleaning staff wear a white coat as soon as they enter the hospital. Anthropologists working in hospitals have examined the historical use of white coats by doctors and the symbolism that they carry (Agic 2012, Mol 2002). They serve to reinforce a demarcation between patients and staff, between the keepers of the knowledge and the ones that depend on them. In the GNH, this hierarchy is strongly expressed.

Altogether there are between 55-60 patients in the hospital at one time, although it is hard to maintain an accurate count since bystanders and patients often go hand-in-hand and some rooms are occupied by whole families. For example, a young female schoolteacher with chronic renal failure resided in the first floor for some weeks accompanied by her mother, who received treatment for her arthritis at the same time. They were visited frequently by the mother's husband, a chubby man in his fifties who stayed in the hospital overnight to undergo naturopathic treatments to decrease the risk of diabetes.

Altogether there were up to one hundred people residing in the hospital during my stay.

I was told that there is a long waiting list of patients wishing to undergo treatment in the GNH and so my research was accompanied by the guilt of knowing that I was occupying a room that could have been used by one or more desperate patients on that list. Since the GNH specializes in renal failure and is the only one of its kind that combines Naturopathy and renal failure as a specialty, it has achieved a solid reputation both inside and outside of Kerala and some patients travel a long way to be treated there. Although the GNH specializes in renal issues, it is by far not the only disease dealt with there – on the contrary, the list of medical conditions is as diverse as in any other Naturopathy hospital: psychological problems, obesity, diabetes, cancer and orthopedic problems.

The daily routine of this hospital becomes clear after a few days. At 6:00 AM patients receive a beverage called *capi* (a Malayalam word for coffee), consisting of herbal ingredients such as cumin and *jageery* (a sweetener). At about 7:00 AM breakfast starts consecutively on the corridors of each floor. The patients leave their rooms with their plates, collect the items and then return to their rooms to eat. The kitchen staff follows lists in notebooks to make sure that each patient gets exactly what the doctor has prescribed. This takes quite some time, as the woman who distributes the food has to check and recheck with her list, while the patients queue to wait for their turn. In the morning there are *puttu* (steamed tubes made out of crushed rice), *doshas* (South Indian pancakes), and several curries produced from vegetables and *ragi* (a type of millet). All dishes are produced without the aid of technical equipment, salt, sugar, oil or spices. Being used to South Indian spicy, oily food, it was quite an unusual experience. In order to achieve this *"completely natural preparation,"* in Dr. Jyotsana KS's words, the kitchen staff works in three shifts, starting at five o'clock every morning. They grind and mash ingredients by hand, cut and steam vegetables, roll out dough, and pick, chop and mix herbal leaves into pastes with their hands and wooden or metal tools with maximum efficiency. An electric grinder would destroy the natural healing power of the ingredients, according to the kitchen staff.

After everybody has had breakfast and cleaned their plates, at 8:30 AM the medical assistant begins his rounds to measure blood pressure. Results are entered into a chart and later transferred into the patient files that Kalyan Ulpalakshan carries on his rounds. Thirty minutes later, at 9:00 AM, Kalyan Ulpalakshan, Dr. Jyotsana KS and the medical assistant begin their official rounds. They walk through every room of the hospital to assess the patient's state of health through a very short conversation. Kalyan Ulpalakshan takes a quick look at the file, asks the patient about their current medication and the progress of the treatment and sometimes examines them physically. Normally the patient or bystander asks few questions, but if they do, Kalyan Ulpalakshan or Dr. Jyotsana KS take the limited time they have to answer. The answer mostly ends in an admonition to be patient, since Naturopathy is a slow process. The medical assistant's task is to report the blood pressure taken earlier and to make notes in the patients' files. Even with 55-60 patients staying regularly in the hospital, some of whom are not in the room when the doctors visit and have to be sent for or returned to later, the whole process only lasts between one and two hours.

Agic (2012) explains what daily rounds in the heart transplantation wards of "his" allopathic hospital looks like.

> The head nurse is the first one following the doctors, pushing the cart with patient files, mobile computer station, medicines, and various para-phernalia. This cart is one of the most important tools in the nurses' work. She is followed by a second nurse, an assistant nurse, and often also a couple of nursing and medical students. During the round work the medical staff visits all the patients in each room of the ward (ibid:307).

This "round work" consists of three phases, according to Agic: First the anam-nesis, where doctors inquire about the subjective experience of the patients, then the physical examination, followed by a conclusion and the provision of information. This scenario is in principle performed by the staff at the GNH. In the late morning between 10:00 and 11:00 AM there is an additional serving of special food, pastes and potions for medical purposes, as illustrated in Figure 7.

This mixture consists of a combination of raw vegetables such as carrots and beetroots at the very back, green herbal leaves ground into pastes in the front, and a variety of juices made out of vegetables, fruits and herbs. When I snapped this picture, I had hoped for detailed information about the ingre-dients of the liquids. I spent hours next to the treatment assistant in order to find out which kind of patients received which kind of medicated liquid or vegetables. However, it took me more than a week and the help of a female English-speaking patient named Abha to convince the treatment assistant to explain the substances of each pot. Although Abha grew up in this area of Kerala and all of the vegetables and leaves used in the concoctions grow locally, it took her further inquiries to understand the treatment assistant's explanations. She dictated to me the Malayalam names of the plants, which I subsequently gave to my assistant Indu for further research. Indu finally discovered many of them

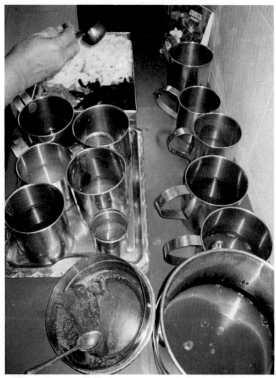

FIGURE 7
*Late morning serving of food,
pastes and potions in the* GNH

on a website about ayurvedic remedies. Others, however, were never identified by Abha, Indu or myself. According to the treatment assistant, each herb has its own significance and ascribed properties: There is, for example, a mashed fruit called *koovalam*[2] that is used by the patients and treatment assistants against diarrhea, fever and uropathy. There is also *cherula*,[3] a kind of water lily, said to be a diuretic and a cure for kidney stones. Barley gruel is served and used against gastrointestinal irritation. For high blood pressure and uropathy, the ground leaves of *njerinil*[4] are provided. The smashed and attenuated *karuka* fruit[5] is served for its antioxidant and antimicrobial effect, and ground *thazhuthama* leaves[6] act as a diuretic, expectant and laxative and are generally used against renal calculi, asthma and liver diseases. All of these herbs

---

2　Bael tree or lat.: aegle marmelos

3　Lat.:aerva lanata

4　Puncturevine or lat.: tribulus terrestris

5　Also called coromandel gooseberry, carambola or simply star fruit

6　Lat.: Boerrhavia diffusa

and fruits are similarly used in Ayurveda and less commonly in Unani, where they are ascribed the same healing properties against certain diseases. These plants grow locally and thus their healing properties are certainly not a secret in Kerala. Some of the patients at GNH know about the healing power of the pastes and fruits they are prescribed, though that does not necessarily mean that they are able to identify them. In the view of the GNH, herbs and fruits do not belong to the category of medication. All natural food has healing properties and here special foods are sought out in order to enhance the patients' recovery. This becomes most obvious by the fact that bystanders and outsiders are excluded from this form of prescribed food. When asked about the herbal preparations, Dr. Jyotsna KS explains:

> Here we don't have ayurvedic medication at all but we use the extract of certain leaves of the plants like *tulsi* juice and seeds. It's not Ayurveda; it's really different from Ayurveda. We have the plants in Thrissur itself; somebody collects them for us.

In her mind, the fact that the herbs and seeds are not processed in any way proves their difference from how they are used in Ayurveda.

Patients queue with their plates and cups in order to receive their individualized combination. Normally they receive a mixture from three or four pots on the treatment assistants' table. Most patients do not bother to ask or make an effort to remember the constellations of their ailments or prescribed food.

From 10:00 AM to 12:00 PM treatment takes place in the form of massages, special baths, mud packs, and wet packs on the stomach or legs. Red lights are commonly used against different types of pain. Sun baths are regularly used and one can observe patients standing outside the hospital and turning different parts of the body towards the sun. Patients are sent to their treatment area for mud baths, while smaller applications such as water treatment on the legs are implemented in the rooms. The treatment is quite complex and can vary daily for every patient. Unfortunately, it is not easy to keep an accurate record of the specific treatment administration for 55-60 patients all receiving individualized treatment in different locations in the hospital. Between seven and ten therapy assistants are involved in the administration and implementation of treatment every day.

Treatment plays a major role in the patients' healing, according to the doctors at GNH. Water applications in particular are said to be very effective in combating chronic and acute renal failure. Dr. Jyotsana KS expressed their importance more than once by asking me, as a German medical researcher and resident, if it would be possible to put them in contact with a Kneipp hospital in Germany in order to conduct further research on renal failure. She wanted to conduct a joint study on the method of water applications.[7]

At 12:00 PM lunch takes place in a similar manner to breakfast. Kitchen staff serve the patients their individual food items according to the instructions on their lists. Again it takes up to one hour until all patients and some bystanders have received their lunch. Afterwards, patients are free until 2:00 PM. Most of them use this time for relaxation, sleeping, chatting with each other, watching TV or receiving visitors. Although exercise is highly recommend by the hospital staff, at this time it is simply too hot to go for a walk. Following this, two additional hours are planned for the individual treatment of the patients.

At 4:00 PM, the medical assistant heads for another round of blood pressure measurement, but this time she only checks the patients whose rates were conspicuous in the morning. Kitchen staff deliver a snack in the form of fruits, pastes, and herbs, similar to the one in the morning. Again it is strictly tailored to the particular needs of each patient and not intended for bystanders or other healthy outsiders. At 7:00 PM dinner is served individually according to the lists. In the evening at 7:30 PM, the two doctors and the medical assistant perform another round through the rooms in order to talk to the patients one by one.

At the GNH doctors work closely with allopathic medicine, treatments and diagnostic methods. Patients are regularly sent to a lab for blood tests; doctors decide about the specific foods and treatments on the basis of these results. For example, if a renal patient has a creatine level of more than eight mg/dl[8] or shows serious symptoms like swollen feet or vomiting he or she is immediately sent for dialysis in order to stabilize their condition. In addition to that emergency plan, it is important to note that many patients take allopathic medication alongside their naturopathic treatment in the hospital. This is not handled as a secret; on the contrary, the medication's mechanisms of action and possible side effects are discussed during the rounds with the doctors. Patients are sometimes even sent to an allopathic doctor in order to receive the correct additional medication for their illness if it cannot be treated fast enough in the naturopathic hospital – for example, to combat dangerously high blood pressure. However, in these instances patients are advised to keep

---

7   Unfortunately, as it turns out, in Germany research on renal failure is not in the hands of naturopathic practitioners but is tightly linked to allopathic treatments and medications, and foremost to the practice of kidney dialysis.

8   Creatine is a by-product of the protein metabolism circulating in the blood and is excreted by the kidney. The higher this level is measured in the blood, the worse the kidney function is. The standard value is 0.8–1.2 mg/dl.

the fact that they are under naturopathic treatment quiet due to the bad reputation of Naturopathy within Allopathy. Apparently, in the past some allopathic practitioners have refused to treat a patient living in the GNH, arguing that naturopathic treatment as it is handled in the GNH would undermine the success of allopathic treatment.

The method of treatment that GNH advocates and has been implementing for the past thirty years cannot be found in educational books; the doctors at the GNH have established their special combinations of remedies through their experience and ongoing experiments. Blood tests in the lab enable them to trace the detailed progress of the patients and their health status and thereafter adapt their treatments. These experiments are not seen to be finished or regarded as a fully-formed treatment theory but are still in the process of evolving. The process reflects the GNH doctors' great interest in the scientification of their practice. Their main objective is to expedite research into water treatment for renal failure in order to legitimize their practice and carry it forward professionally. Unfortunately, they lack the financial means for such research on a broader scale.

In terms of outside networks, the GNH does foster links with other naturopathic practitioners in Kerala: Dr. Ramakrishnan, who maintains a hospital specializing in orthopathy in Tirur, was once employed at the GNH. Dr. Madhavan, chief physician at the MNCC in Bakkalam, was treated by Prof. Ulpalakshan – Kalyan's father – for his tonsillitis some decades ago. Notably, the GNH management declines opportunities to work with other naturopathic institutions.

2   Nature Life Hospital, Kozhikode

The Nature Life Hospital (NLH) in Kozhikode, located next to the civil station and four kilometers away from the town center, is one of the first hospitals founded by Jacob Dr. Vadakkanchery. It is managed by his wife Soumnya, who studied psychology at Kozhikode University. The building itself is not on the main street but on a quiet side road. It is in quite good shape and well-maintained. It has two floors for living, a ground floor with group rooms and consulting rooms, and a huge rooftop terrace. Altogether there are 25 rooms for patients and their bystanders; sometimes whole families reside here. Generally every patient brings at least one bystander, who also stays in the hospital. Like all psycho-nutritional hospitals, NLH serves a considerable number of outpatients and daily visitors, who sometimes stay overnight. This includes counseling and treating people who would describe themselves as completely healthy on the basis that they lack any disease or do not have any physical complaints. Some are curious about Naturopathy, while others want to express a local patriotism but are not sure what that would mean in terms of nutrition. There are a great number of political activists who travel for various kinds of campaigns and decide to stay with like-minded people on their way.

The space here is a relatively open one. On average there are between forty and fifty people staying in the NLH. On the ground floor there is the dining room, referred to as the "diet corner," and the kitchen where three women prepare the meals and snacks. In addition, one can find Soumnya's office, a library and a consultation room, separated from the hall only by saloon doors and therefore not insulated to ensure the privacy of conversations. Patients normally avoid these rooms unless a doctor or staff member invites them for a counseling session. However, it still happens that patients or visitors decide to have a private conversation in the consultation room or discuss a book in Soumnya's office. On the other side of the building there is a large common room with a TV and a table for *carroms*, a popular table board game whose rules lie somewhere in between billiards and table shuffleboard. This is where the lectures and the evening games take place.

The rooms have attached bathrooms and are fitted with rudimentary furnishings – a table, bed and small cupboard. The beds lack mattresses, and the thin sheets hardly cover the wooden boards of the bedsteads. Since the laths have some distance in between them, they are not necessarily pleasant to sleep on especially during the first nights. As was explained to me, lying on mattresses is unnatural and disturbs the recovery of the body. There is no AC in any of the rooms and no intention to add it, since air conditioning is considered to be unnatural. However, all the rooms are equipped with an electric ceiling fan.

Three people are mostly referred to as doctors by each other as well as by the patients: Soumnya, her husband Dr. Vadakkanchery, and Dr. Balakrishnan Nair. The latter is an elderly man and volunteer worker, who used to be employed with the railway and has now completed a short course of education in Naturopathy. He is primarily an autodidact, and spends a lot of time reading and lecturing about what it means to live a life in tune with nature. In addition, there are three women who work in the kitchen and seven helpers – five women, two men – for the treatments. Soumnya's father is also employed in the hospital; he is concerned with administration and accounting and does not provide direct patient care. Soumnya lives in the hospital most of the time while her husband, Dr. Vadakkanchery, occasionally visits and sometimes stays for a while. Dr. Nair uses a room on the first floor. The treatment helpers, who are not from Kozhikode, share sleeping places on the first floor as well.

There are no dedicated rooms for treatment and it takes place in the patients' rooms, in the corridors, or outside in the courtyard. Every day, approximately ten outpatients come for counseling either from Soumnya or from Dr.

TABLE 3   *Daily schedule for patients at NLH*

No.	Activities	Time	Location
1	Wake up alarm, Enema detox	5:00 AM	Rooms
2	Measurement of blood pressure, sugar, etc.	6:00 AM	Prayer hall
3	Herbal juice	6:10 AM	Prayer hall
4	Yogic *kriyas*	6:30–7:30 AM	Open air/terrace, Yoga hall
5	E.N.T. wash	7:30 AM	Open air/front courtyard
6	Sun bath	7:45–8.30 AM	Open air
7	Breakfast	8:30 AM	Diet corner
8	Rounds (Doctor)	9:00–10:00 AM	Respective rooms
9	Treatment	10:00 AM–12:30 PM	Respective rooms
10	Herbal juice	10:30 AM	Diet corner
11	Lunch	12:30 PM	Diet corner
12	Relaxation – Eye pack	1:30 PM	Yoga hall
13	Study class (lecture/CD)	2:00–3:00 PM	Prayer hall
14	Herbal juice	3:00 PM	Prayer hall
15	Treatment	3:00–5:00 PM	Respective rooms
16	Sun bath	5:00–6:00 PM	Open air
17	Dinner	6:00 PM	Diet corner
18	Night gathering	7:15–8:30 PM	Prayer hall
19	Retire/sleep	9:00 PM	Room

Nair, whose office is next door. Rooms for inpatients cost 550 rupees per night including the special diet and treatment. According to the staff, this is at cost price.

In the NLH everything works according to a structured schedule that is posted in every room; during the daytime there is almost no available time for extra activities (Table 3).

Patients are expected to wake themselves at 5:00 AM. Some of them receive an enema or perform their own enema. From then on, most of the activities take place in a social frame. The patients meet in the morning at 6:00 AM for their blood pressure measurement. This is followed by a short group prayer and the consumption of the morning herbal juice, which consists of a vegetable called *kumbalanga* and *koovalam*[9] leaves, in the common room – here called the prayer hall. *Kubalanga* (a type of bottle gourd) is meant to encourage the activity of the bladder and the kidneys while *koovalam* leaves protect against diabetes by strengthening digestion. As both prevention and cure, all patients are expected to drink juice. Subsequently, the patients collectively ascend to the roof terrace for the Yoga *asanas*. Those who cannot participate for health reasons or do not want to do Yoga themselves stay on the rooftop in the shade to observe, comment and praise the progress of the Yoga practitioners. The management of the NLH invites different Yoga teachers for these sessions. For example, during my stay in the NLH there was a woman from Russia, traveling through Asia, who met Dr. Vadakkanchery on an airplane from Thailand to India. Since she has always been interested in Naturopathy and is a Yoga teacher by profession, she decided to stay at the NLH for a couple of weeks and to teach daily sessions of Yoga and sometimes meditation.

The ENT (ear, nose and throat) wash and the sun bath both take place in the front courtyard. The patients share the three popular newspapers that arrive every morning, *Malayalam Manorama*, *The Hindu* and *Mathrubhumi*, and discuss their thoughts about the treatment and the content of the newspapers. Breakfast is served at 8:30 AM and like all the other meals takes place in the diet corner, where small tables are placed together to form one big table around which all of the patients gather. When the meal is ready, one of the kitchen workers rings a loud bell. The atmosphere is cheerful; patients warmly welcome newcomers while everybody consumes the well-arranged fruit or vegetables plates (Figure 8).

The food served is generally the same for everybody. One has the choice between raw fruits (bananas, coconuts, watermelon, papaya, or grapes) and vegetables (cucumber, tomatoes, or carrots) for three meals per day, and patients usually select fruit in the mornings and then vegetables for the other two meals. Some overweight patients are fasting and only consume juice, which is also prepared with the help of a kitchen machine in the diet corner. During the meal the patients debate the taste of the fruit and their desire to alternate a very spicy fish curry once in a while. The discussion often turns towards the "best" or "most traditional" dish they can prepare and patients compete – men as well as women – about the recipes of these dishes. The conversation normally concludes in agreement that naturopathic treatment is fantastic due to its positive effect on weight loss.

---

9   Bael tree or lat.: aegle marmelos

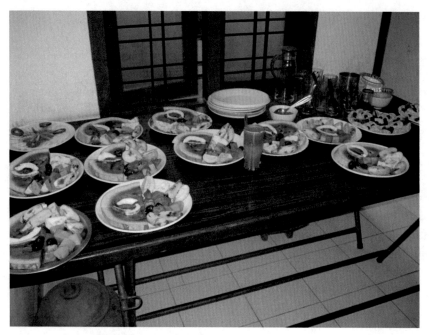

FIGURE 8   *Fruit plates arranged in the NLH*

After breakfast, there are rounds through the ward. At least one of the doctors visits all of the patients to discuss their well-being, lab results or possible
changes in the treatment. The doctors wear their normal everyday clothes for
that. The process takes a fairly long time, during which the patients' doors are
usually left open and some curious patient or bystander might follow the doctor to the next patient and join the conversation about disease, nature cure
and the right way of living. Especially when there are visitors from far away,
such as myself or anybody else with an interest in Naturopathy, Soumnya, Dr.
Vadakkanchery or Dr. Nair take plenty of time to explain the cases, the treatments and, if necessary, translate. Every patient has a file that is created when
they arrive at the hospital in which the prescribed treatments are listed.[10] This
file is not carried around by the doctors during their rounds; instead, they
almost always know their patients and the particulars of their cases and, if not,
they will listen to the case story from the beginning. The individualized treatments are recorded in simple charts in the file in order to help the treatments
assistants to implement the right modalities.

---

10   The case history file can be found in the appendix

For male patients, treatment is carried out mainly in the corridor. There, they sit or lie next to each other, chatting or joking, while they enjoy a cold eye pack for relaxation or some other prescribed treatment. For women or for patients receiving treatments on delicate parts of their body, these therapies take place in the corridors or outside in the courtyard. However, for practical reasons, water treatments are implemented in the patients' rooms or in the attached bathrooms. One can often see the treatment assistants dragging huge metal tubes through the corridors for hip- or spinal baths. Since some of the treatments require undressing, female patients mostly stay in their rooms for treatment.

After their first round of treatment, patients gather again in the diet corner for their juice at 10:30 AM. It is made out of gooseberries, an incredibly sour fruit rich in vitamins, especially vitamin C. Afterwards, there is time to relax. Patients utilize their free time to play *carroms*, watch TV, sleep or finish their morning conversations. Everybody meets again in the diet corner for lunch at 12:30 PM.

After lunch there is an hour of relaxation before the lecture begins in the common room at 2:00 PM. The lecture is normally held by Dr. Nair. At the beginning of each lecture, he counts all the patients present, and sends someone to gather any missing ones who have gone for a walk or fallen asleep. The lectures generally focus on educating the patients about food and the body, and are peppered with local-patriotic statements about Kerala's ideal climate, and its sweet, perfectly-grown fruits. In contradiction to the basic rule of the Nature Life branch to "keep everything very simple," these lectures are filled with specific rules about the consumption of food, and the patients learn about proteins, vitamins and carbohydrates, as well as their use and abuse. For example, patients are taught that liquids must be taken at least half an hour before having food and that the latter has to be chewed a certain number of times before it can be swallowed. Patients learn about the functions of their body, the digestive and respiratory systems and how to deal with them in a "natural" way. Dr. Nair summarizes the ideology of the education lessons: "*The most important matter is to have a clear mind and sattvic food.*" These lectures are interactive, meaning that Dr. Nair regularly asks participants questions in order to make sure they are listening, and he offers an opportunity for questions and discussion. I was told that if Dr. Nair is not in the building, one of Dr. Vadakkanchery's DVDs is shown on the television.

At 3:00 PM, patients receive another herbal juice in the diet corner. This time it contains *njerinil* (puncturevine) water, used to activate blood circulation. It is produced as a powder in the factory managed by the NLH branch in Ernakulam. This drink and the one in the morning are the only two exceptions to the rule of only eating raw fruits. Following this, another treatment session commences and patients either go back to their rooms or gather in the corridors in order to wait for the assistants. Patients who are supposed to undergo sun baths and those who are chatting with the sun bathers meet in the courtyard.

At 6:00 PM the bell rings again and the fruit and vegetable plates for dinner are served. The night gathering at 7:15 PM is an obligatory event. Every evening the patients meet in the common room, put chairs in a circle and play various games together under the guidance of a treatment assistant. This resembles a group therapy session since the treatment assistants even think of role-plays where patients are asked to act out different social situations. The atmosphere here is very cheerful, and patients are encouraged to demonstrate different talents – singing songs from their childhoods, showing dances they learned at school or acting out pieces of a play. Foreigners in particular are required to produce some sort of "cultural heritage" daily in order to satisfy the curiosity of the other attendants. The three doctors do not take part, but the kitchen staff and the treatment assistants normally attend the gathering. The day is finalized with the routine of singing the national anthem together. Shortly after 9:00 PM the activity dissolves and the patients move back to their rooms for an early bedtime.

A strict routine keeps patients involved in social activities throughout the day. The doctors and other hospital staff join them as often as possible and chat with them about health and disease as well as other diverse topics, ranging from communism to road-building policies. Frequently Soumnya and Dr. Vadakkanchery invite a group of patients to their house for lunch or dinner. In these gatherings, the food consists of vegetarian, not-so-oily dishes, freshly prepared by one of Soumnya's relatives or by Soumnya herself.

Although allopathic data from the patients' biomedical history is collected at the beginning of their treatment and organized in the file, the hospital staff refrains from conducting blood tests on the patients. Only if a patient explicitly wishes to track the progress of the healing is he or she sent to a lab nearby. However, allopathic diagnostic methods are not scheduled for the patients and their wish is normally carried out with an echo of profound disapproval from the hospital staff. Patients are strongly advised to stop all their allopathic medication as soon as they enter the hospital. There are some exceptions though, such as psycho-pharmaceuticals, for which the NLH doctors advise a continuation of the medication at a lower dose until the body adjusts to living without it. Most of the patients adhere to these regulations, and those who do not try their best to keep their violation of the regulations secret. The NLH maintains strong links to other institutions led by psycho-nutritionals, predominantly the other NLH hospitals and smaller hospitals in the area. The collaboration consists mainly of the joint planning of events, such as health camps, or in the exchange of patients – for some patients, another location may be more practical depending on where they live.

3   Three Methods of Treatment

Examining the daily routines of the GNH and the NLH is important in order to understand the paths of these two hospitals. Taking into account the practices at both institutions, I distinguish three different forms of treatment on an analytical basis.

The first form is tangible and substance-related. It has two main characteristics: 1) it includes a haptic (tactile) experience, either of temperature or material or both, and 2) it is set within a specific framework designed for this treatment and accomplished with the help or guidance of a treatment assistant. Most of the treatments elucidated in naturopathic textbooks are designed on the basis of the five *panchabutha* elements and fall into the latter category, with the exception of meditation and fasting. Although both of these latter exceptions occur within a specific framework and are guided by assistants, they can be defined more specifically by the lack of a haptic experience. Substance-related treatments are quite unusual for most naturopathic patients in their daily lives: The use of bathtubs, massages, sun baths, mud packs or even Yoga *asanas* are not part of their normal schedule.

The second form of treatment is nutritional therapy – the diet. It is the naturopathic treatment that both the public and some practitioners associate most with Naturopathy, even to the point of many people assuming that there is no treatment in Naturopathy other than nutritional therapy.[11] Although every hospital employs a specific idea about the perfect timing and contents of the diet, the idea of food being the main cause of intoxication, referring back to Kuhne's assumption in the 19th century, is universal in naturopathic hospitals.

The third type of treatment is some degree of psychological integration proposed by the directorate of the hospital through their daily schedule or overall ideology. I refer to this method of social integration as "psychological" due to the previous education of most naturopathic doctors, which leads to the use of psychological methods such as counseling and behavioral therapy.

---

11   In the naturopathic units of other hospitals, such as ayurvedic or allopathic clinics, the
        only treatment offered is nutritional.

Naturopathic education is an integral part of this category since it always takes place during group sessions and is meant to stimulate group interaction.

These three types of treatment are not exclusive and self-contained; in fact, there is such a wide range of possible mixed variations, flows and transitions between them that a "pure" form of treatment only exists on an abstract level.[12]

The daily routine of the GNH, the professional hospital, reveals that its main emphasis is on nutritional therapy and applied substance-related therapies. Psychological integration plays a minor role, if any at all. Nutritional therapies lie at the fore of the treatment. According to the ideology of the GNH doctors, the main obstacle to living a healthy life is the intake of wrong, "unnatural" food. Rules about its intake are strict, well-organized, and individualized to the specific needs of each patient. Single food items are seen to have unique medical effects and so due to the patients' varying conditions, each person receives a different diet plan. Three principal meals and two snacks provide the basic therapy for patients and are designed to effect all medical changes: cleansing the blood, decreasing creatine and blood pressure, burning unnecessary fat cells and reducing nausea. The use of medical drinks during the twice-daily snacks plays a major role in this scheme. Thus, in contrast to the NLH, the diet plan at GNH is personal, individual, exclusive and non-transparent.

Substance-related therapies are administered for two hours daily. Every patient undergoes a somewhat confusing full set of these therapies every day, one type in the morning and another type in the afternoon. Patients normally wait in their rooms for the treatment assistants, not knowing exactly how many and what kinds of treatments they will receive that day. The effects of these therapies are not explained in detail to the patient and are therefore difficult to reconstruct. Apart from the treatments employed with mud, most applied substance-related treatments take place in private in the patients' rooms. Some materials, such as smaller bathtubs, can be easily transported and purchased in the hospital itself, but usually there is no great interest on the part of the patients to continue these treatments at home. I only met one patient with renal failure who bought a tub for his daily hip bath and wanted to transport it to his home in Tamil Nadu.

---

12   Yoga *asanas*, for example, can have a strong communicative character if they are seen as integrative activities where patients support each other in both physical and psychological ways. Substantive treatments such as mud packs can be accompanied by bonding and counseling activities by the treatment assistant. Due to the sensory and interpersonal element of substance-related therapy, it can never be seen as merely a mechanical application of materials. Likewise, meals can be promoted as a common activity for sharing experiences or they can be taken alone in the patients' rooms, sometimes even at different times.

Education with regard to naturopathic theory and practice does not take place in a formal way. Even in face-to-face interactions, doctors rarely have time to explain their motives to the patients, since they are overworked and must care for such a large number of patients. Overall, doctors, medical assistants and the treatment staff have a very formal relationship with the patients. Encounters are restricted to the daily rounds, blood pressure measurement and the application of substance-related treatments. The patients, on the other hand, enjoy frequent interaction and create strong bonds with each other as a consequence of their close physical proximity and shared experience of illness. However, patients who do not wish to establish contact with their co-patients are not pressured by the organization of the daily routine, common meals or even by the staff in the hospital. In my experience, there were several patients who completely avoided leaving their room. One of them was a Muslim teenage girl whose mother, staying with her as a bystander, was so overprotective that the other patients spent hours guessing what disease she had – or even what she looked like – since nobody actually ever saw her in the corridor. Her mother collected her food and instructed her to stay in the room. At the NLH this would not have been possible.

Considering the shortage of time that doctors and medical staff are confronted with at the GNH, efficiency and professionalism may seem like a logical consequence of the development of this specific naturopathic hospital. Another reason may be that in the market of medical systems treating serious and life-threatening diseases such as renal failure, cancer and others, professionalization is often deemed necessary to compete with rival institutions. For example, in order to "scientificate" their practice, doctors experiment with food and applied substance-related therapies. The outcome of these experiments are monitored in patients' blood tests. This explains the necessity of regular blood samples. When asked about *panchabutha* and the allocation of treatments, Dr. Jyotsana KS explained to me:

> We are dealing here with real diseases. The five elements and their treatments we surely learned in our education and this is the theory. In practice people are suffering from serious health problems and we need to give them relief without the theoretical background. They do not need to know all this to experience healing.

Their ambition to start randomized trials, preferably with an institution located outside of India, corroborates this attempt to establish an authorized and permanent position within the medical pluralism existing in South India.

Some of these emphases and practices contrast to those at the NLH, the psycho-nutritional hospital. Using the three modes of treatment as a basis for analysis, it becomes clear that there is an emphasis in the NLH on nutrition and psychological-integrative activities. The most remarkable point about the daily routine in this hospital is the fact that the patients are kept busy most of the time and incorporated into social activities. A group dynamic is created and often compared by the NLH staff to the atmosphere found at ashrams. Communication and understanding are seen as the key to health and therefore privacy is deliberately limited. The community and its social interaction comes to the fore; patients with less-developed social abilities are identified by doctors and through individual discussions, and they are then integrated into the group. Doctors and their treatment assistants are no exception to this; indeed, they make a great effort to establish a conversational rapport with all of the patients to make them feel comfortable on an informal basis. The fact that doctors do not wear any kind of uniform is intended to reduce hierarchical structures beginning at this visual, symbolic level. Patients should see the doctors as one of them and feel comfortable and encouraged to understand their disease, their body and the way that healing can be achieved. Doctors and staff also communicate with patients in their off-duty hours, and friendships and joint excursions between doctors and patients are commonplace. Doctors generally have a welcoming attitude and try to integrate newcomers by introducing them to the rest of the group. Dr. Vadakkanchery in particular is very concerned about the personal well-being of the patients and his wife Soumnya uses her psychological training to meet the patients' counseling needs.

The regular, obligatory and formal meetings at NLH, such as the lecture after lunch and the evening gathering, urge the patients to confront themselves while supporting each other. Singing, dancing and joking with one another are highly encouraged and welcomed, as are discussions about diet and treatments. On special occasions such as health camps, the management invites musicians or friendly, musically-talented psycho-nutritionals to visit, who help to establish a group dynamic by coaxing and animating the patients to sing popular faith songs. Patients already follow a regular schedule that does not vary significantly, so they have frequent opportunities to share their experiences during the group meals or treatments. Even though patients in both hospitals hail from a variety of backgrounds in the multi-religious and multi-caste and -class state of Kerala, the psycho-nutritionals endeavor to minimize these differences by focusing on humanistic, egalitarian values.

Nutritional therapy is the second most important emphasis in the NLH. Group meals containing raw vegetables and raw fruits are distributed to the patients three times per day. The most striking fact about this diet is that everybody receives the same meal. The staple ingredients are coconuts and bananas, the fruits that Malayalis refer most to when they express a local patriotism.

There are only a few deviations from this rule: for example, newcomers receive fat-free dishes with rice and steamed vegetables in the beginning in order to get used to the NLH lifestyle, and extremely overweight patients are put on a juice or water fast to facilitate rapid weight loss. For the purposes of simplicity, meals are intentionally kept basic. Thus, their preparation is easy to remember and replicate at home. All of the ingredients are obtainable locally; if they do not grow in one's own garden than the fruit shop next door should carry them.[13] However, during the health camps, the NLH management sometimes serves dried rice and steamed vegetables since they are afraid of frightening off curious visitors at the very beginning. Psycho-nutritionals are convinced that by eating raw and locally-sourced food, the patient receives whatever he or she needs to strengthen the body's ability to heal itself. The prescribed diet is common, impersonal, universal (in other words, everybody receives the same foods), and transparent.

Substance-related treatments are regularly used at the NLH for most kinds of diseases. However, doctors do not expect the patients to be able to remember or to implement their specific treatments at home after leaving the hospital. This is the reason why patients are never given full explanations. In addition, they are not part of the content of the lectures. Massages are not conducted at all, or at least there were none during the period of my fieldwork. The theory of the *panchabutha* elements and the allocation of treatments is also not an issue addressed by doctors or hospital staff. The health camps organized by psycho-nutritionals usually do not employ applied substance-related methods. Instead, psycho-nutritionals invite political speakers, hold joint Yoga sessions, and share "natural" food with the participants. Thus, on the whole, substance-related treatments are seen as an additional aid or complement to nutritional therapy and psychological integration, the two treatment forms that are given the highest priority at NLH.

In sum, although an organizational framework is used in order to structure the daily routine, the emphasis of the treatment goals is on social interaction as an integrative part of the healing process. Since many of their treatments are alike, individual diseases are less in the spotlight than the general well-being of the group.

---

13   This is also the reason that apples are not served: they have to be imported from Karnataka and thus belong to the category of luxury, non-locally-sourced items that must be avoided.

4   Conclusion

There are multiple ways of interpreting the theories and fundamentals of Naturopathy. Even while belonging to the same medical system, the GNH and the NLH promote different practices, especially in terms of defining what it actually means to "live naturally." The social practices of these two hospitals are an example of the heterogeneity of naturopathic treatment in Kerala. It is instructive due to the particular similarities and differences in the approaches both hospitals maintain in administering treatments.

Both hold a strong focus on nutritional therapy. This is not surprising as food is constitutive to the movement's self-conception. Ingestion is the most powerful bond one can establish with natural living. This focus distinguishes both naturopathic hospitals from allopathic treatment centers. The second unifying quality of both institutions is their structured, sophisticated processes and daily routines which turn both sites into highly complex organizations separated from the rest of the world: hospitals as naturopathic spaces.

The way this otherness is constructed, however, differs between the professional and the psycho-nutritional naturopathic hospitals. In the GNH doctors have tightened their focus on applied substance-related methods. These methods remain mostly unexplained, but are standardized and constantly validated with blood tests in order to improve and fine-tune the results. Nutritional therapy is a question of highly-individualized, prescribed food with special healing substances. In the GNH, medical knowledge is not transmitted to the patient (or the ethnographer).[14] It is restricted to the site and to the persons that professionally deal with it: the doctors.

In the psycho-nutritional NLH the situation is different: Here the main focus of therapeutic treatment is on the psychological integration of the patients and their bystanders, the doctors and personnel, as well as all other politically-motivated people spending time in the hospital. The education received by patients in lectures and the integrative style of handling the treatment itself is intended to bring them closer together and to foster the development of a group dynamic in which patients can encourage each other to adhere to the treatment. A key characteristic in this hospital is the importance of non-individualized nutritional therapy. While nutrition is of highest relevance in the treatment of the patients, it carries the same importance for everybody in the hospital: Everybody – patients and non-patients alike – receive the same diet.

---

14   The GNH was the only hospital where backgrounds were regarded as confidential. In all other professional hospitals, I received detailed or at least semi-detailed information on the individual treatments of patients, as well as their background profiles.

The right kind of food is not so much a substantial form of medicine, but rather it is an integral part of the naturopathic way of live. Overall, the focus in NLH is on the communal aspects of hospital life. Individual diagnostics and treatments of diseases – and therefore the use of a clinical gaze – take a back seat. A main focus of every kind of treatment is simplicity and transparency. Continuous explanations by doctors and their assistants about the purpose of accomplished treatments are meant to transfer the medical knowledge to the patients so that they can take it out of the hospital into their own living environment.

It becomes evident when comparing the everyday life in naturopathic hospitals with ethnographic materials from allopathic hospitals that Naturopaths cumulatively adapt the complex processes of allopathic hospitals and therefore employ the allopathic clinic as a model. Therefore biopower in the form of the establishment of specialist knowledge becomes an integral part of everyday life in the hospitals. As a specific example of a professional hospital in Kerala, the GNH does so on a far greater scale than the NLH, a hospital led by psycho-nutritionals. However, while practitioners in the GNH employ further techniques such as the administration of individualized substances or the restriction of medical knowledge to the site in order to construct a naturopathic space, the naturopathic doctors of the NLH deliberately counteract these techniques, thereby turning the hospital into a political site that aims to educate patients as independent human beings.

CHAPTER 5

Naturopathic Actors: Between Ideology and Practice

The monsoon season had arrived as my friend and I spent another day in a naturopathic hospital. He acted as my driver, introduced me to numerous practitioners and political activists, translated, organized, explained and interpreted, collected magazines, arranged appointments for interviews and located someone who could repair my computer. He and most of his relatives had been in the naturopathic field for quite a long time and he was thus a respected member of the community, well-versed in the rhetoric and daily hospital routines. We were in full action for the whole morning. For lunch we had a plate of raw food, just like the patients and the practitioners. Due to the heavy rain and several power cuts, everything was happening more slowly than usual. We were very tired in the evening and had gathered a great amount of data that still had to be classified. The hospital provided us with a number of patient files that we planned to sort through that same evening. *"Shall we have a Biriyani and continue with those files later? I am starving,"* my friend asked. *"How can you be a Naturopath and have Biriyani?"* I wondered. Biriyani is a delicious, spiced rice dish that in Kerala normally comes with ingredients such as vegetables and/or chicken and by all means is not naturopathic. *"I am not sick,"* he replied in a lower voice, *"and we will go to a place far from here."* I agreed.

∵

In contrast to allopathic practitioners, Naturopaths usually attach great importance to the ideological side of their practice. They consider Naturopathy not only to be a medical system, but a conviction that permeates every layer of everyday life. Psycho-nutritional Naturopaths told me repeatedly how important it is as a political statement. Consumption becomes crucial to all aspects of life, from the daily nutritional intake to the selection of clothes, means of transportation, and products for bodily hygiene.

Psycho-nutritional Naturopaths in South India often claim the normative scope of everyday life. For many outsiders this scope appears rather extensive: Life decisions such as marriage options, career plans, and place of residence are supposed to match up with a naturopathic lifestyle. However, many Naturopaths do not lead a completely consistent life. As the ethnographic vignette at the beginning of this chapter indicates, there are exceptions. Exceptions of social rules often explain more about the particularities of the normative context of a community than the rules themselves. In order to investigate such meaningful inconsistencies, this chapter starts by analyzing Naturopaths' personal convictions and motivations, as well as the frictions within the lives of practitioners in naturopathic hospitals. How important is a naturopathic ideology in their professional lives? Is this ideology constitutional for their choice of profession, e.g. to become a doctor? Or do doctors learn the ideology and begin to consider it important during their training or even in the context of their everyday practice in the hospital? What is the role of the professional site of their practice?

There are a great number of people involved in the daily care of patients in Naturopathy hospitals. The hospitals of all of the medical systems in India employ helpers to administer medical treatments and to care for the patients. Naturopathic hospitals in particular use treatment assistants and kitchen staff, whose backgrounds and prospects form the focus of the next part of this chapter. What role does naturopathic ideology play for them in the selection of their profession as well as in their everyday hospital life? The final part of the chapter addresses the issue of social stratification in naturopathic hospitals. The naturopathic ideology is crucial for everybody involved in the movement, and the role of the hospital is pivotal for its construction as a naturopathic space.

1   How to Become a Naturopathic Doctor

The number of planned naturopathic colleges has increased in recent years. Even Kerala, until now a state without naturopathic colleges, plans to offer future BNYS courses in at least two locations,[1] and professionalized naturopathic treatment has become increasingly mainstream. Psycho-nutritionals for their part are also gaining followers, advocates, and general popular acceptance, not least through their involvement with other social movements. However, there are significant differences between the motivations of naturopathic professionals and psycho-nutritionals.

---

1   One of them is planned by Father Philip Neru, who is currently the head of the department of physiotherapy in Thiruvananthapuram, also known as Trivandrum, the capital city of Kerala in the very south. Another is planned by a married couple close to Kozhikode who are also very active in INYGMA. They have already opened a biennial Masters course in Yoga and Natural Therapies in an institute affiliated with the University of Kozhikode.

Two main reasons for pursuing professional Naturopathy education predominate in my sample. The first reason is to fulfill the expectations of their family. In particular, children of the middle class in Kerala – as well as children from working-class families – are put under pressure to either study engineering or medicine, since both of these degree courses and the subsequent profession hold very high prestige in the region and increase the overall status of their family. Studying medicine also guarantees the sought-after title of "doctor."[2] As doctors are seen to embody good character and strong moral and social values, this profession is particularly appreciated as a career choice (Zola 1972).

One female post-graduate (PG) student in the Universal Good Life Ashram (UGLA) pointed out to me:

> I actually wanted to become an engineer but then my father said, I should go for BNYS because my brother is already an engineer. My father was always very much interested in Yoga so he was also interested in BNYS. I was not so much interested in going for a medical profession but he gave me those two options so I chose BNYS. At least I have chance to go abroad and teach Yoga and Naturopathy at other places with this education.

The fact that her parents are able to pay for a college education indicates at least a middle-class background, where children are obligated to aim for a career at the same level as their parents or higher. Although there is a quota for castes in the medical exam, social climbers are very rare in the medical field. Out of all my interviews with BNYS degree-holders or candidates, only one candidate from a so-called "backward caste" admitted to having been granted special entry by the directorship of the first College in Hyderabad in the 1970s.

Some BNYS doctors confided to me that their family had actually planned for them to study allopathic medicine. If their medical grades were not high enough to train as an allopathic doctor, they still retained the option to choose from other health-related fields such as Ayurveda or nursing – the latter still having the advantage of the title and the prestige of working in a medical field. Naturopathy is a comparatively new and developing field. For this reason

---

2 Anthropologists Osella and Osella (2000) and other social scientists (e.g., Mathew 1997) have ratified the high importance of education in Kerala. Parents and relatives support each other in order to finance courses and exams for their children – the latter sometimes more than once until their child has passed. This is the only opportunity to help their children work either as engineers, in the medical field, in more financially-lucrative positions in a Gulf country, somewhere else abroad or, if they are lucky, in Kerala itself, where well-paid jobs even for high-qualified people are rare. Schoolchildren experience an immense pressure to fulfill the high educational expectations that their social environment places on them.

alone, students interested in medicine consider it to hold more potential prospects for promotion in comparison to a well-established field such as Ayurveda or one of the other state-supported systems of medicine.

The second reason that students cite for deciding to study professionalized Naturopathy is that they believe in it. Naturopathy appears to them as being very "Indian" and not as commercialized as Ayurveda or one of the other AYUSH systems of medicine. They mentioned their affinity towards Yoga as a motivation for studying Naturopathy and Yoga at college. For those students who had had some prior experience with Naturopathy and thus claimed ideological motivations for initially pursuing education in the field, those reasons center on the non-invasive nature of treatment. Naturopathy is viewed as *"not having side effects," "not being as cruel as Allopathy,"* or *"having a holistic approach [that] is not only physical healing."*

However, as it turns out, over the course of the research I discovered that the principal reasons for studying Naturopathy are, at least in the beginning, mostly pragmatic – many of these young scholars began to consider a naturopathic profession because of family pressure. In most cases, the ideological conviction only arrived later. Most of those students already had a personal or family experience with Naturopathy. Very often a relative, convinced of the healing power of Naturopathy, might hold a naturopathic degree or had undergone naturopathic treatment. As a PG student from a naturopathic hospital in Thiruvananthapuram explains:

> I became a Naturopath because in my family history there are many practitioners of Naturopathy. My father's brother [has] a garden and he has a naturopathic hospital close-by and my father's brother's son also, he is the first BNYS doctor from Kerala. He is in the government hospital in Ottopalam. And he was [the] principal in my college.

Another doctor from the GNH reports similar experiences:

> My father was an allopathic doctor; he had diabetes and started Yoga. Before that he was on allopathic medication for years but it did not help him at all. I remember about my father that he did a lot of Yoga and in the end he controlled his diabetes with it, then he gave Yoga classes for asthma patients. After we had seen the success, he sent me to Mangalore to study Naturopathy on a professional level. That is where I first found out about it.

One degree-qualified doctor from the National Institute of Naturopathy (NIN) in Pune points it out very clearly:

It was an accident you can say. I completed my 12th standard, then I had to opt for a professional course. I was not knowing anything about Naturopathy but I didn't want to study in Kerala. I wanted to go out of Kerala and of course my favor was always towards science subjects like medical or paramedical or something like that.

He further explains that his family, after long deliberations, decided to place him in a College for his education because his grandfather had once undergone treatment. He comments how studying Naturopathy finally convinced him:

In the first year I was not really convinced but in the second year I saw again some cases which I had worked with in the first year. And they were cured. We were not exposed to the clinical side in the first year. It was all theoretical classes. And then I saw some cases even one syphilis case and another tough case. I was very interested in these two cases and in the 2nd year we had a lesson [about the] philosophy of nature cure taught by our principal. She tried to explain what Naturopathy is, how diseases are caused and how they are cured. In one class, in one talk, I was totally impressed by Naturopathy. She explained how diseases are caused. Then I understood that it is toxemia [that] is the cause of the disease. And how toxemia generates [a] different level of diseases. We can say it [in] 2 or 3 sentences but it has gone into my heart. And then I understood that it can be cured. That was the initiation I got; as you can say guru-to-disciple sometimes the light comes, and that happened in my second year when I saw these two cases again and they were cured.

These motivations on the part of BNYS practitioners – i.e., having the family pressure of studying something prestigious and or following a family member's conviction – are applicable to all naturopathic students and degree-qualified doctors I met. They constitute a new generation of young naturopathic scholars who do not believe that self-education can provide the full depth of information that Naturopathy holds.

In the case of non-qualified practitioners, their career path development is not at all as homogeneous as those of the BNYS doctors. This becomes most obvious when grouping together all non-degree practitioners who treat or advise patients and call themselves doctors of Naturopathy. Not all of them would self-identify as psycho-nutritionals; some also work in health centers or private health institutions. Although their backgrounds may differ considerably, it is possible to identify one similarity as the lowest common denominator:

they are all located in the wider field of social service or social health care. They became familiar with Naturopathy either through this social service or because of an experience with illness themselves. They learned about Naturopathy autodidactically, mainly through networking in the naturopathic field in Kerala and its surroundings.

Dr. Vadakkanchery, for example, was educated as a social worker and worked in this profession before he became involved with Naturopathy and, modeling Gandhi, started his own "experiments":

> I cut my tea and coffee and non-vegetarian food which was very tough at that time, 30 years back, because I lived in a coastal area, a fish[ing] village near Ernakulam, so I belong to a traditional Christian community. It was very tough to stop non-vegetarian, fish, meat, egg, then there were severe oppositions from every side, family, friends, neighbors, community. Then to stop drinking tea and coffee is also difficult because as a social worker I have to visit various houses, many houses every day and I have to travel with my friends and unable to eat from home, always outside so everybody offered tea and coffee. So saying no to tea and coffee when you visit a house is very impolite.

Through NGOs and colleagues in the field of social work, he learned more about naturopathic ideology and treatment. He started advising friends and other help-seekers about health issues. These activities were financed through selling *japi* (a naturopathic replacement for coffee, containing cumin and the sweetener *jageery* but no caffeine) to several *kadi* (a Malayalam word for snack shops). In 1997 he opened a restaurant in Ernakulam in order to provide "*normal people a chance to have natural and healthy food every day.*" This restaurant became very popular and soon he started to concentrate more heavily on treatment facilities and finally opened his first hospital next to Ernakulam. In this hospital he treated "*hopeless cases with great success*" and it continued to expand. For Dr. Vadakkanchery, Naturopathy was included in his critique of a modern lifestyle but constituted only one element of his ideology.

The former head of the department of psychology at the University of Kozhikode, Dr. John Baby, also an associate of the psycho-nutritionals, was drawn into the practice of medicine in general because of his family background:

> I did not even take any drug in my whole life, maybe for some ten rupees but that was thirty or forty years ago. My father died at the age of 103, he was here in this house. He had never taken any drugs in his life, like my

mother, she was 97 when she died. They taught us all these principles with health. They were followers of these local remedies, Ayurveda; he was a qualified traditional ayurvedic doctor, my father, qualified in the traditional sense, a *vaiyda*.

Eventually, through the influence of some of the early pioneers, mainly C. R. R. Varma and Mr. Radhakrishnan in Tamil Nadu, Dr. Baby developed an interest in naturopathic treatments. The most fascinating aspect of Naturopathy for him was its simplicity – the fact that only a relatively small amount of knowledge, and of course a lifestyle change, is needed for the treatment. Although Dr. Baby comes from a working-class Christian family, he married a Brahmin Hindu woman. It was a love marriage and Dr. Baby converted to Hinduism for her. At that time, in the 1970s, this was such a scandal that even the media reported about it. Nowadays it fits more comfortably into the egalitarian worldview of psycho-nutritionals.

Another example, Mr. Kurian, is an adviser of Naturopathy in a treatment center in Kottayam, founded by C. R. R. Varma two decades ago. His work consists of supporting outpatients in leading a life in tune with nature. Since the possibilities for applied substance-related treatment methods in this center are very limited, Mr. Kurian is restricted to making suggestions for improving diet in terms of "localness," rawness and freshness. Mr. Kurian also provides psychological advice to his patients in order to help them lead a more harmonious family life. He formally studied sociology and community development but since he could not find employment in those fields, he had started working as an electricity clerk when he came in contact with Naturopathy. By chance some of Varma's books fell into his hands. Mr. Kurian, already well-versed in Gandhi's visions from his studies, became completely absorbed by Varma's ideas. When Kurian's son fell ill, he met Varma at a center in Kottayam and received quick, successful treatment for him. According to Mr. Kurian, his son has not been sick since that incident. After this experience, Kurian decided to give up his secure employment with the Kerala railway and stayed in the center to promote Naturopathy and to advise patients seeking help, where to this day he shares his knowledge and convictions. Mr. Kurian is an active member of a group in Thiruvananthapuram that engages in a variety of social activities. His latest project is promoting zero budget farming, a development of organic farming that works with self-sustaining local methods. Supporters of zero budget farming promote the usage of only natural and local fertilizers for farming, whereby they refer to products that can be allocated to one of the *panchabutha* elements (see Palekar, unknown date). Mr. Kurian, for example, uses Indian cow dung as fertilizer for the plants in his garden. He is trying to set an example of practicing subsistence agriculture, for now limited only to his family but he has plans to introduce this to the whole of Kerala.

A last example of non-degree-holder motivation is a Christian priest from Ernakulam who is now the head of three hospitals and an author of several books and magazines about Naturopathy. He experienced an illness that was cured by Naturopathy after a long period of suffering:

> I had some difficulties with my lungs, asthma, headache, fever, cough, heaviness, tiredness and I was always using medication, English medicine or ayurvedic, then – somebody introduce[d] me to nature cure and I started practicing it. After 15, 30 and 60 days most of the sickness was cured and then I began to learn and teach others and started this center in 1981. From 1978 onward I was practicing, that means using for myself and for others who were sick and told them to come and start practicing. Then it was very good result so I started this center and I learned all the natural methods to cure, we included prayer also, prayer means meditation, it was very useful. We have come across all types of sicknesses like cancer or heart attacks. I went to many centers to learn, because in the beginning no universities were teaching, only private academies, so I went to Shivanda Yoga Ashram in Thiruvananthapuram. I stayed there 1 month and they gave a very good class of Yoga *asanas*. It was 1983, I came back and sent my sisters so we have 65 sisters in 3 nature cure centers, Ernakulam and Maharashtra. I met Varmaji[3] in Ernakulam where he was giving instruction for sickness. Varmaji was consulting patients about food mainly.

After this priest's experience with illness he decided to undertake a short training in Naturopathy, which in the early 1980s was only available in Hyderabad. Through his own healing experience he became convinced of the benefits of Naturopathy, changed his lifestyle and felt compelled to spread the message. He sent his sisters for training; some of them even attended BNYS courses. Additionally, he was in charge of the funds donated by the community, and therefore able to build hospitals and purchase the basic equipment. Thanks to a church exchange mission, the priest once traveled to Bad Wörishofen in Germany in order to learn Kneipp's water treatments first-hand. For this priest, Naturopathy is a necessary part of Christian education, since helping sick community members is a core Christian value. In his practice he gives medical

---

3   The priest is referring to C. R. R. Varma. The ending "ji" is commonly added to names in India to convey respect.

treatment at no charge to those who cannot afford it. His medical choice fell on Naturopathy because, according to him, Jesus did not use any medication for healing his disciples and the Bible gives examples of Christians healing themselves with naturopathic applications such as water.

Naturopathy for psycho-nutritionals and other non-degree-holders in this study is basically a second career; all of them do have some kind of formal academic background. They learned the applications primarily by self-education and networking, and chose to practice Naturopathy because they believed in it.

2   Being Private – Being a Naturopathic Doctor

There is pressure for psycho-nutritionals to live according to their principles outside of the hospital in order to be positive role models for their audience. Unfortunately, however, this lifestyle is not very practical for social gatherings or sharing everyday life with those who are not like-minded. Of course, it depends upon the individual follower of the psycho-nutritional movement as to what extent they live on raw fruits and wear non-imported, preferably self-made clothes, and variation exists. I did meet a small number of highly idealized psycho-nutritionals and other non-degree-holders who drive their families crazy by demanding that they live strictly on local, raw or semi-processed food, and by requiring them to avoid unnatural cosmetics and walk to their respective jobs or schools every morning instead of taking the bus, no matter how far or how uncomfortable the weather. Others do not have a family and practically live an anchorite life. A very small number of idealistic Naturopaths are lucky to be with a like-minded partner by choice and therefore able to implement most or at least some of their ideological values. However, these people were the exceptions and not the rule.

I used to spend quite some time with one psycho-nutritional – I will call him Mr. Kutty here – who was involved not only in hospital work but also in the political movement and in the organization of health camps. When he left after the health camps and other events he used to give me a ride in his car since we lived fairly close to one another. He regularly ordered his driver to take him either to a *hotel* (the local word for a small restaurant) or to his house to have dinner, although he had already participated in the raw food dinner at the respective event. At midday he enjoyed tea and served his guests snacks such as *laddu* – an Indian sweet snack consisting of chickpea flour, sugar and plenty of ghee or oil. When they invited guests for the evenings, Mr. Kutty and his family served delicious, full vegetarian meals, typical for the region and equivalent to the ones prepared by my host family, who had never been engaged in any naturopathic activities. At times, Mr. Kutty invited me to social gatherings with other psycho-nutritionals and political activists where they served large vegetarian meals with cooked food, spicy curries and boiled rice, discussed future plans of action and wove networks with like-minded people in the social or political fields. Some of these gatherings took place in the dining hall of a hospital, but excluded outsiders such as patients. It was not a rarity for a hospital staff member to serve the food (and have cooked it) and then devour the leftovers in the kitchen. Some gatherings at private houses even included the consumption of non-vegetarian items such as fish or even chicken.

Mr. Kutty was rather surprised that these practices seemed contradictory to me. He told me that he would certainly not have integrated me into his private life if he had not already given up on turning me into a *"real Naturopath,"* or if he had known that I had any kind of health problem. *"In general,"* he said, *"it is better to have raw food all the time. But in daily life this is hard and not practical."* He added that living a life completely in tune with nature would not be very convenient for his adolescent daughter, who has to be taken seriously by her friends and teachers. His wife would also not agree with *"turning our family meetings into raw food festivals."* However, he swore by the fact that every time he or one of his family members or colleagues became sick, they would fast strictly for several days on water or coconut milk and then eat only raw food until they felt better again. *"When somebody is sick, there is no other option,"* he explained. They would never take any kind of other medication since this would be akin to a complete poisoning of the body and they would probably never recover from the side effects. Mr. Kutty added that he had not taken any allopathic or ayurvedic medication since he was around twenty years old and started to believe in Naturopathy.

This matter is handled in a similar way by degree-qualified doctors. Most of them do not eat at their place of work, in the hospital itself, but rather disappear for lunch and dinner. One Muslim female PG student living in a hospital in Thiruvananthapuram admitted that she is strictly on a naturopathic diet as long as she stays in the hospital and eats with the patients. She is convinced that this provides motivation and a positive example for the patients. But as soon as she goes home for the weekend or a holiday, she and her family consume meat curries, which she enjoys very much. She is also convinced that the raw and natural diet is only necessary in the case of sickness.

During my research I had an insightful experience while I was under treatment in a naturopathic hospital in the countryside. This time I was strictly following the orders of my doctors since I wanted to experience the realities of being a naturopathic patient. Furthermore I wanted to rid myself of a minor skin disease that had afflicted me for several years. For three weeks I had restricted myself to raw food and was practicing Yoga daily for three hours. I sweated in steam baths and was wrapped in banana leaves on the hospital roof in the midday sun. One afternoon I walked out of the treatment center and was returning to my room – having just received a very pleasant massage – when a car stopped next to me. Somebody rolled down the tinted windows. I recognized the driver as an employee of one of the wealthier patients in the hospital, and a young female patient sat in the passenger seat. Two of the hospital's young BNYS doctors sat in the back. They asked me to join them and as soon as I got into the car and we drove around the corner, the two doctors opened bags of sweets, offering them to everyone in the car. We drove for about half an hour through the countryside; everybody was cheerfully chatting until we stopped by a *hotel* in one of the villages. I felt perturbed when they invited me to have "real" food at this place, since at that time I had decided to give naturopathic treatment a serious chance against my skin disease. In the end I dismissed their offer. When I gave them my reasons they told me, "*but you are not that sick, you do not need to be on raw food all the time!*" Before we left, the driver took another plate of food to go and told us that this food was for the hospital director's wife, who had asked him privately to collect it for her. My refusal to eat the restaurant food that night came with the consequence that all of them were constantly worried that I could whistle-blow to the director of the hospital, and they never asked me to join them again.

These two anecdotes are perfect examples of the rifts and inconsistencies occurring in the biographies of naturopathic practitioners. On the outside, both psycho-nutritionals and professionals constantly endeavor to be role models for their patients. However, taking a closer look at their everyday lives reveals that, with some minor exceptions, both groups view naturopathic food and treatment primarily as a way of healing disease, at least for themselves. This relates to their personal lifestyle choices and whether they want to be socially included or just enjoy the taste of a spicy curry occasionally. However, they all distinguish between the image they display to the external world and the personal life that they lead, a distinction that does not strike them as contradictory.

3   People from the Village: Treatment Assistants and Other Associates

One of the main differences between naturopathic and allopathic hospitals is the lack of nurses in naturopathic hospitals. Instead, each naturopathic hospital employs a number of treatment assistants responsible for implementing the prescribed treatments as well as kitchen employees who prepare the food for patients. Newcomers and outsiders to naturopathic hospitals, however, sometimes refer to the former as nurses until they have a better understanding of their tasks.

Agic (2012) describes nurses as the *"flow of information"* in his allopathic ward, the connecting piece between patients and doctors. Nurses collect information, keep the files up-to-date and inform the doctor about the condition of the patient and the patient about the results of his examinations and further treatments. They take blood samples, bring them to the lab, measure patients' blood pressure and administer their medicines. Treatment assistants in naturopathic hospitals do not carry out any of these tasks. In Zaman's (2004, 2005) ethnography of an orthopedic ward at a Bangladeshi allopathic hospital, he calls nurses *"frustrated voices"* (among others) who are overworked, underpaid and enmeshed in bureaucratic obligations at the expense of being able to devote more time to patient care. This is also not the case for naturopathic treatment assistants. Street (2014) describes the nurses in "her" hospital in Papua New Guinea as engrained with social knowledge that is seen in sharp contrast to and hierarchically below the medical knowledge of the doctors. Treatment assistants, kitchen stuff and receptionists in naturopathic hospitals do not hold such a position. The tasks assigned to treatment assistants in naturopathic hospitals do not necessarily include caregiving or active listening, as the above-mentioned literature suggests for nurses. Treatment assistants are not available to patients "on demand"; instead, they arrive only at the time of their treatment shifts. Their primary task is to execute the applied substance-related treatments prescribed by doctors. In practice this means smashing and preparing the herbal drinks together with the kitchen staff, crushing mud for mud packs, brushing cloths with mud, setting up tubs for the spinal- or hip baths, preparing red lights for pain relief in muscles and using these appliances on the patient. Treatment assistants also help in the hospital kitchen or even assist in cleaning if necessary.

Figure 9 depicts two female treatment assistants in their daily tasks; one is brushing mud on a cloth (NLH), while another is distributing food (GNH).

Working as a treatment assistant is a job that requires training, but there is no standardization for it. The NLH branch is the only venue where a formal training has been established, most recently in Ernakulam, in order to disperse treatment assistants to various in-need hospitals and health camps in Kerala. This is the reason why treatment assistants in NLH hospitals live in the hospital itself: they are transferred wherever there is a need for helpers. Those who are regularly transferred are young and unmarried. In all other naturopathic

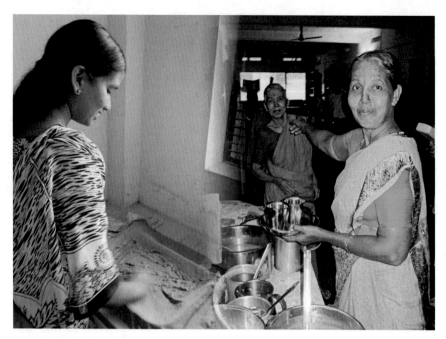

FIGURE 9   *Two female treatment assistants*

hospitals, treatment assistants are recruited locally and trained for the specific needs of the hospital. They come in the morning, help in the hospital usually for two treatment shifts, and go home in the evening. Most of them are female, middle-aged, with children at home and without any other education, helping their household to survive. There are also a small number of men working as treatment assistants for male-only treatments that women do not receive. Some treatment assistants have previously worked in other nursing jobs, looked after children or cared for the elderly, and are therefore experienced in caregiving. Some of them have even received naturopathic treatments before. They get a job in the naturopathic hospital mostly by recommendation and are instructed for about two months until they can work independently.

Since I hardly met any treatment assistants with fluent or even basic English, my conversations with them were limited to the women's group treatment sessions through other female patients who acted as interpreters. Although we were urged not to talk too much in order to allow the treatment to work better, while we were lying with mud-soaked cloths wrapped around our chests or other parts of our bodies, it was often the only chance for me to find out about their lives in this intimate group of half-clothed women. My own treatment assistants always told me how much they enjoyed their jobs; they liked to be surrounded by people, and to chat and laugh with them. They enjoyed the calm atmosphere in the hospital. Doctors hardly had any reasons to be angry with them since in a Naturopathy hospital there is no time pressure for giving the patients their treatment. Patients are normally not in imminent danger of deteriorating or even dying. Although they receive only a minimum salary, they explained to me that they considered their jobs stable and not too stressful. Applied substance-related methods are not urgent and so both patients and treatment assistants enjoy having chats during or mostly after the treatment. All of the treatment assistants I met were cheerful, friendly and welcomed my company during their treatment rounds to show and even teach me the different kind of methods they were practicing.[4] When asked about their prior knowledge, most of the assistants said they had not known about Naturopathy before they came to the hospital. As soon as they became accustomed to their new jobs, however, they began to like the idea of people being cared for in such a slow and relaxed manner. I heard many stories about treatment assistants sending their sick family members for naturopathic treatments or conducting them at home, since they had become convinced of their efficacy. Thus, in their own families, these assistants provide access to a health system that other family members would likely not encounter otherwise.

Rajata's Story

Rajata, a young woman in her early twenties, works as a treatment assistant at the NLH in Kozhikode. She comes from an Ezhava family residing close to Kottayam. Her father once participated in one of Dr. Vadakkanchery's health camps in Kottayam to seek help for diabetes, from which he had suffered for over ten years. In this health camp he learned about the role of diet in the fight against his disease and became accustomed to eating raw food at least twice a day. Later on he went to an NLH in Ernakulam in order to deepen his knowledge and live completely without any medication. He greatly enjoyed his stay and recommended the NLH course for treatment assistants to his daughter, who was then 17 years old. When I met Rajata, she was in the first year of training in the program. She enjoyed her job and felt very honored to work for the health system that had freed her father from medication. At that time she shared a room with a few girls working in the NLH kitchen, and sent part of her monthly salary of 6,000 rupees back to the family household in Kottayam.

---

4 There was a constant misunderstanding about my role: treatment assistants either thought I was a "full patient" and did not need to know more about the correct handling of the treatment or they thought I was there to learn different treatment techniques. So it happened that I even learned how to do different kinds of oil massages for back pain.

Rajata has wide-ranging and high-responsibility tasks to contend with in the hospital since the administration was convinced of her personal dedication from the beginning. She especially enjoys the evenings in the NLH. As she told me once, it fills her with gratification to see how people can blossom in a positive group atmosphere. According to her, the positive attitude that develops from the shared evenings has a strong effect on the rehabilitation of the patients' bodies. Rajata is not aware of the fact that none of the people she refers to as doctors in the hospital have a medical degree. When I tried to talk to her about the education of her colleagues she simply shook her head and said: "*I know that they are healing, I see it everyday so they are doctors.*" When Rajata is sick herself, she tries to avoid all forms of processed food and – if necessary – fasts for a while.

Veena's Story

Veena is from Taliparamba, a small town close to Kannur in the North of Kerala. She is 47 years old and has worked at the Mahatma Nature Cure Center (MNCC) – a hospital founded by a non-degree holder that now employs BNYS doctors – for four years, some twenty minutes by bus from her town. Veena has three children and a grandchild on the way. Her husband is a bus driver, and they had suffered from financial troubles in the past. About ten years ago when all the children were old enough to take care of themselves in the afternoons, the couple decided that it was necessary for Veena to contribute to the household expenses. She began working nearby in better-off households and even farther away in Kannur. She cleaned houses and cooked for other people until one of her employers told her about the MNCC and the fact that they were looking for treatment assistants. Veena applied because she hoped to be able to reduce her commuting time. At the time of the interview she was working on the female ward in the MNCC, brushing mud on cloths and putting them on different parts of the patients' bodies. In the mornings and evenings, she is responsible for applying water packs to the chests of female patients in their rooms, who are fasting in order to stabilize their blood circulation. Additionally, she is trained in massage for female and sometimes even male patients. She related to me that one of her favorite aspects of the job is that she encounters people she otherwise would never have met – patients from other parts of India seeking health care and even foreigners like me. Veena was so curious about my European life that she even spent extra time after work trying to get more information about the marriage system in Germany. She confided to me that she definitely wants to stay at the MNCC because she thinks that her employers here are the nicest she has ever had. Every time her daughter experienced trouble during her pregnancy the doctors in the MNCC looked after her and helped her to feel better.

The kitchen staff have a similar status as treatment assistants in naturopathic hospitals. They comply strictly with the doctors' instructions for preparing food according to the patient files, plus an additional amount of food in case unexpected patients and companions show up. They are also recruited locally, work in different daytime shifts, do not have any higher education, and leave the hospital in the evening. The kitchen staff is all female. In some hospitals such as the MNCC, a number of general helpers are employed to work in the kitchen, take care of general cleaning and bring water and juice to the rooms of fasting patients.

Every naturopathic hospital hires cleaning staff to clean each patient room daily. Furthermore, every naturopathic hospital employs a number of men and women to work as daytime receptionists. They are responsible for bureaucratic matters such as answering the phone, registering new patients and taking care of the accounts. These receptionists are usually from the local area, and unmarried receptionists might even live in the hospital. Most have received a basic education as accounting clerks or secretaries, and unlike the other hospital employees, they often speak other languages such as Tamil, English or Hindi, which they use to communicate with the many patients coming from outside of Kerala.

In the hospital's social hierarchy, there is no status difference between treatment assistants, kitchen staff and general helpers. All are referred to by both patients and doctors as "women from the village" or "people from the village," accentuating their localness and non-worldly wisdom. Generally, they all follow the instructions of the doctors.

Treatment assistants enter Naturopathy in quite a similar way to degree-doctors: Because of a family or employer recommendation they consider naturopathic service as a career option. The reason they decide to stay, though, is quite different: Once familiarized with Naturopathy, both groups become convinced that they are doing a service not only for their own financial stability but also for mankind. The conviction clearly follows the practice. The difference between the motivations of treatment assistants in professional and psycho-nutritional hospitals are minimal, with the exception that treatment assistants tend to stay overnight in psycho-nutritional hospitals, while most of the treatment assistants in professional hospitals leave after their shifts have ended.

4   The Social Stratification of Naturopathic Hospitals

Kerala is a highly structured and complex society. Different levels of castes interweave with layers of religion and create a social hierarchy that varies

regionally. Despite the dissolution of these structures at least in an urban context through increasing mobility and new job market options,[5] this emerging
equality is still somewhat superficial. The specific local features of a shifting
stratification have yet to be discussed and examined in strictly local circumstances and are only valid for a very short period of time. On a day-to-day basis,
women remain generally responsible for all household tasks. Nowadays they
are not only the main performer of domestic services but are also expected to
pursue a proper education and contribute to household finances. Children
born into a traditionally disadvantaged group still experience inequality and
deprivation on a structural level, despite the compensatory effort of the government. Members of the different religions in Kerala are still involved in
different types of turf wars, especially legal issues concerning property or land,
and access to positions in the civil service and public administration.

Psycho-nutritionals present themselves as people who have a strong sense
of morality, adhering to values such as family solidarity, and they maintain an
egalitarian and humanitarian view of the world. Woman's double burden is
strongly decried by psycho-nutritionals as a negative trend. Equally, the strong
stratification of Malayali society has been a hot topic addressed by psycho-
nutritionals. An integral part of the "come a patient – return a doctor" slogan is
the idea of the empowerment of the individual – which stands in contrast to
the predominant class and caste system in Kerala. One would expect that the
inner composition of the psycho-nutritional movement would stand in clear
opposition to the hegemonic structure of society.

However, regarding practices and structures of psycho-nutritional hospitals
and health camps, little effort is made by the hospital administration to counteract stratification among the hospital employees themselves. Instead, psycho-
nutritional hospitals basically reflect the social structure of Malayali society.
Although psycho-nutritionals generally have not received a formal medical
education, all of them do have either academic training or a middle-class background. They are clearly in control of the treatment administration as well as
the overall processes in the hospitals (and also in health camps). On the other
hand, treatment assistants mostly come from underprivileged groups. They are
strictly dependent on the instructions of the doctors and do not usually have
any formal education outside of the hospital; this also applies to kitchen workers or cleaning staff. The hospital staff have no prospects for professional
advancement or gaining greater treatment responsibilities. Stratification only
dissolves on an informal level, where friendships between patients of diverse

---

5   Osella and Osella (2008, 2000) are among the pioneers examining this new pattern of social
     organization in Kerala.

backgrounds and treatment assistants or even doctors are encouraged. Women are generally underrepresented within the psycho-nutritional field. During my research I only met two women, one being Dr. Vadakkanchery's wife and the other one a Muslim woman, who are involved in the psycho-nutritional cure, actively speak for themselves in public, advise patients on lifestyle issues, and treat their diseases. Generally the number of Muslims is very low, while the proportion of Hindus active in the field of psycho-nutritional cure is comparatively higher. Most psycho-nutritionals in my sample originally come from a Christian community although some have distanced themselves from religion in general and are even active in the atheist movement in Kerala. Whether this is due to the geographic site of my research or to some other factor is a question for future research. The fact remains that psycho-nutritionals, who as a group feel strongly about social equality, have developed a strong social hierarchy within their established spaces.

On the other hand, professionals as a group are not necessarily concerned with matters of societal equality or the empowerment of women and other underprivileged groups. This is clearly reflected in their hospital structures, where authority and status differences between treatment assistants, other staff and doctors play a major role in the daily routine. However, in my experience the proportion of women in degree colleges or who are educated, hospital-employed doctors is at least 50%. Further, a number of professional naturopathic hospitals are managed by women. Although a shift towards the feminization of formally-educated medical practitioners can also be observed in other countries, the difference between psycho-nutritionals and professionals in this matter is remarkable.

5 Conclusion

The various actors in the naturopathic setting in South India have diverse motivations for pursuing Naturopathy and for maintaining their commitment to it. Initially, BNYS holders generally decide to consider Naturopathy because of their family members' ideological convictions and wishes for their choice of occupation. For most of them, becoming a doctor is central to their choice of profession. The type of medical system itself is less important and depends on the possibilities at the time they enroll at college. On the other hand, non-degree-holders usually make the decision to pursue Naturopathy based on their own convictions. In almost all cases Naturopathy is a second career in their lives. Often, a significant personal experience preceded their "enlightenment," such as an illness that could not be cured by other medical systems. In both groups there is an implicit separation between Naturopaths' private and professional lives. Most prefer a socially compliant lifestyle and use food as a medicine in case of sickness but not necessarily as a preventative measure.

When considering the hospital as a naturopathic space, this distinction makes perfect sense as the division of professional and private life relates to the conception of space. For the doctors, ideology as well as illness belongs to the hospital. Curing patients requires ideology as well as a change of diet. However, outside the clinic doctors' private lives do not require this ideology. When they are not sick their dietary choices remain unrestricted.

Aside from the patients (whom I shall describe in the following chapters), the remaining significant actors in the naturopathic hospital are the treatment assistants as well as the kitchen workers. They are recruited for their jobs from the local villages. Like BNYS doctors, most started their occupation with no ideological commitment or motivation. Most had no prior knowledge of Naturopathy. However, after an initial entry phase of indifference toward the medical system, their attitudes towards Naturopathy changed as they began to believe in its principles. They pragmatically implement naturopathic treatment methods and diet in the event of their own or a family member's illness.

For psycho-nutritionals, the hospital constitutes an ideological space. As described in the previous chapters, psycho-nutritional naturopathic practitioners stage it as the non-hierarchical and egalitarian site by ensuring that everyone eats the same food, sleeps on the same kind of bed and does not have unequal access to luxury items such as air-conditioned rooms. Thereby they attempt to empower the individual patient to become their own doctor. However, in taking a closer look at the overall hospital organization, it becomes clear that psycho-nutritionals grapple with the reality of providing medical services in a competitive health and labor market. In this process of bureaucratization, it seems difficult and simply not pragmatic to fully implement this egalitarian ideal in the institutions of psycho-nutritional Naturopathy. Furthermore, an egalitarian division of knowledge and power by the psycho-nutritional doctors does not take place. Both are intended to be transferred by the doctors exclusively to the patients, but not to the hospital workers.

What this chapter reveals is a deviation from ideology on the part of actors in the practice of Naturopathy. This makes the naturopathic space ideologically constructed, at least in its delimitation towards professional naturopathic hospitals. Even if ideology precedes psycho-nutritional practice, it is only relevant for the individual doctor but not for the structure of the movement.

CHAPTER 6

The Logic of Labeling: Diagnostics and Naturopathy

Naturopathic textbooks include discussion of diagnostic techniques, such as iridology, Kuhne's investigations of facial expressions and pulse diagnoses (2010 [1917]). In the German naturopathic literature, follow-up exams using the same techniques are described alongside diagnostic applications. Likewise, Indian theoretical literature teaches the same diagnostic methods. However, in all of my experiences with naturopathic practices in India and elsewhere, I have never witnessed practitioners make use of these methods or even refer to them during a patient's hospital admission process or later. During my fieldwork in Indian naturopathic hospitals, the act of diagnosing a patient was not considered to be a central task with accompanying consequences for the remaining hospital stay.

Labeling a patient with a diagnosis is always a complex interactive process of power asymmetries and negotiation in which both the healer and patient are involved (Smith-Morris 2016, Jenkins 2014). Patients' belief systems and explanatory models for pain, ailments or feelings may differ from the normative scales of the particular medical system to which the healer belongs (Kleinman 1980). The healer localizes the patient's symptoms and interprets the latter within the framework of the respective medical system. Both interpretations – the healer's and the patient's – might be conflicting. The situation of competing paradigms and its impact becomes more complex as the differences between explanatory models increase. According to naturopathic theory, all diseases can be traced back to intoxication, which is seen to be caused by unhealthy diet or lifestyle decisions. Therefore Naturopathy is one of the so-called holistic systems of medicine, aiming to heal not only the isolated symptom or single organic cause of a disease but the "whole person" with all of the physical, mental, moral and other aspects.

However, despite its holistic approach, the language and content used by both Naturopaths and patients when talking about ailments and their treatment are biomedicalized. Furthermore, biomedical diagnostic tools such as blood tests are used to create and adapt a treatment plan. This chapter explores the underlying rationale for this hybridization. First, it scrutinizes the ways that diseases are identified and categorized in naturopathic hospitals and the relevance of this process for the patient's social life inside and outside the hospital. In order to understand this social contextualization, it is crucial to examine how patients get involved with Naturopathy in the first place and

© KONINKLIJKE BRILL NV, LEIDEN, 2016 | DOI 10.1163/9789004325104_009

thus analyzing its interwoven relationship with Allopathy allows us to comprehend a patient's choice to pursue naturopathic treatment. Finally, using the example of mental illness, I argue that the way that naturopathic physicians handle the labeling of disease can create new social space for patients.

1   Health-Seeking Behavior in South India

In India, the body, the whole person, and his or her health are seen to be continually produced and reproduced through social interactions between people and their environment (Nichter 2001). An important aspect of caring for one's own health is the act of going to a doctor, even more so than the Western belief that individuals have a duty to be self-responsible and to maintain the self-control necessary to follow a "healthy lifestyle" (Wilson 2010a, 2010b). In light of the range of medical treatments presented in the first chapter, one might ask: how do patients select a treatment from the myriad medical strategies on offer in South India? It is the specific disease that dictates whether one chooses a Homeopath, a Naturopath, a psychiatrist, or a Christian church? Or, is it a question of personal conviction if one considers first the opinion of an astrologist versus an allopathic specialist or an ayurvedic physician?

Several studies have focused on what anthropologists call health-seeking behavior in South India.[1] According to Alex (2010), patients generally adhere to one of two overarching priorities in deciding where and with whom to seek health care:

1.   When pragmatic and logistic parameters are at the forefront (i.e., the local and financial accessibility of a medical system and its practitioners);
2.   When the explanatory models of health, the body or sickness of the respective practitioner coincide with one's own understandings or beliefs.

---

1   Referring to Alex (2010), most of these studies are a follow-up to the introduction of the term health-seeking behavior by Charles Leslie in the 1970s and 1980s. For example, Beal (1976), who studied choices in health matters in South India, came to the conclusion that allopathic doctors are often the first choice of patients living in an urban environment due both to the high prospects of success and their accessibility. Geertsen and colleagues (1975) found that a person's social relations and ethnic origin held more sway in the choice of a medical system or healer. Apart from these ethnographic analyses, quite a number of models for health-seeking behavior have evolved since the 1950s in neighboring disciplines such as social psychology and medical sociology. These models were developed in the context of public health projects that aimed to predict and control the behavior of patients in health-seeking circumstances. A summary of the models can be found in Hausmann-Muela et al. (2003).

Health-seeking behavior in South India depends strongly on context: for example, whether the patient lives in an urban or rural environment, whether they have a family inclination or affinity towards a certain kind of treatment, or even whether they have a medical practitioner as a relative. Other possible factors include the financial means of a patient – for example, health insurance or access to other financial resources. Mobility plays a major role in health-seeking behavior, and whether or not a patient has access to the infrastructure or free time necessary to reach far-flung hospitals or practitioners. In anthropological literature, the term "healer shopping" (Kröger 1983) has become established. The "Indian patient" in particular is considered to make use of divergent medical systems either simultaneously or consecutively in order to ensure the best possible health outcome.

While this study was not directly concerned with the health-seeking behavior of patients in South India and therefore cannot make a representative statement about patients across existing medical systems, the above points apply to most of my interview participants in naturopathic hospitals. Both models introduced by Alex (2010) are true for patients in my sample. All of them visited a healer for their ailments as soon as they could afford it, and considered the act of seeking health care to be more important than attempting extended self-help practices. The chosen treatment generally cohered with their place of residence and degree of mobility. All of them had tried at least two medical options before I met them. The first one was usually Allopathy: when they felt the first pain or irregularity in their body, they consulted an allopathic doctor who sent them to a diagnostic center for further investigation. The order of frequented medical systems was then determined by the local availability of practices – such as Ayurveda or some type of religious healing, depending on the patients' beliefs or preferences. Not a single patient that I interviewed had consulted Naturopathy before that point.

Upon being asked about the healer-shopping patients, one practitioner at the GNH affirmed:

> That is true, in India people move around a lot. If you get a disease you go to an allopathic doctor first. Then let's say about 5% or 8% of the people go to Ayurveda. 2-3% will go to Homeopathy. But most of the patients go to an allopathic doctor first. From there they find out that they don't have a clear remedy for their problem, so they opt for other systems of medicine.

2   **Allopathic Diagnostics and Naturopathic Treatment**

Patients in South India are strongly biomedically socialized. The dominance of allopathic values and models cannot be denied and what a lab technician presents in cold print is both the starting point and continuing reference point for the naturopathic patient – and likewise for the patient of Siddha medicine (Sujatha 2011). Indeed, all patients interviewed had already received a fixed diagnosis by the time they arrived at a naturopathic hospital and a large proportion of them had already sought allopathic treatment. The following excerpt from my transcripts concerning the cases of two patients in a naturopathic hospital exemplifies the interaction between allopathic diagnostics and naturopathic treatment:

> Rounds at a psycho-nutritional hospital in February 2010, my additions in parentheses:
>
> "Patient 1: A man in his late 40s who stays in the hospital with his wife
> Naturopath: (speaking to me) He has chronic tonsil infections. He was using toothpaste before. Toothpaste is very toxic; it will absorb the enamel, all the calcium, everything from your teeth as well as your jaws. He was having difficulties on his jaws, it started bleeding. Now he has stopped everything dental, toothpaste and everything he has stopped; he is using herbal paste only.
> (to Patient 1) Have you ever tried oil? A spoonful of it? It helps a lot, you know. Use pure organic sesame oil, cold-pressed sesame or cold-pressed sunflower, or cold-pressed coconut oil on an empty stomach.
> Patient 1: To drink?
> Naturopath: (to Patient 1) No. Not to drink. You take a spoonful and you swish it in your mouth. It's very effective you know. It cleans the mouth and the teeth.
> Patient 1: I have this bleeding and swelling. What does it come from?
> Naturopath: (to Patient 1) Due to gland enlargement. (to me) You want to see his test results?
> Me: Yes, of course.
> Naturopath: (to me) It's in very medical terms. Technical, very technical. I will explain it to you later (hands me a sheet full of charts).
> Patient 1: But is this swollen gland due to nutrition? What is the cause of the swelling?
> Naturopath Physician: (to the patient) They (allopathic doctors) say some kind of malignancy is there so we'll remove something for further testing and then see how we proceed.

(Patient says something in Malayalam).

Naturopath: (to me) Do you understand what he said? He has this enlargement from there to there. Maybe it extends from this side to this side, but the (allopathic) doctor doesn't know exactly what it is. He gave antibiotics. (He laughs) He had it for six months and it didn't go down. (to the patient) How long have you been here now?

Patient: Four weeks.

Naturopath: (to me) It has reduced now. He is using herbal paste instead of toothpaste. And a special diet. For the first four days only – water diet, nothing else. After that he had pineapple juice and orange juice and all the other days the same diet. He lost three kilograms although he has nothing to lose. He is on full rest, not supposed to go out. No talking, maximum voice rest because he wants to get repaired. He's only getting up to drink something."

"Patient 2: A man in his late 20s who is staying in a hospital room with a 50-year old man.

(Short conversation with the younger patient in Malayalam; both patients speak only Malayalam).

Naturopath: (to me) He is here with his father, and he has BP (high blood pressure). His father also has it (pointing towards the father). It's genetic. They were taking tablets but only one is left, see, he has taken almost all of them. After tomorrow there will be no more tablets for them. Only nature cure. We reduced the dose slowly.

Me: So what does he get here?

Naturopath: (to me) He gets gooseberry paste; its very good for BP. That cools your brain and is good for blood circulation, so BP comes down. And he also gets the diet. He has fruits only. We have very good results with that. He also has renal failure. Doctor told him to do dialysis or transplant. Such a condition he is in! Both kidneys have a very low functioning or no functioning. For that normally you have to do dialysis in Allopathy. As a result of the kidney failure the BP is increasing. The circulation is not good. We cannot try all the treatments because of the blood pressure. All these problems he has. His condition is very complex. Potassium, urea and creatinine have to be controlled. We checked it 12 days back and we have to recheck it after 15 days. And then we know what the differences are, how much he got better. That's how we do it here. There are also some Yoga *asanas* for that."

As Nichter (2002) observed particularly for Gulf repatriates in South India, people are increasingly seeking out allopathic medical diagnoses during times of illness in order to decrease what can be an uncomfortable feeling of liminality. The realization that patients want to have an allopathic diagnosis as soon as possible is the primary reason why Naturopaths do not use the methods of facial diagnosis described in their textbooks, instead relying on the allopathic diagnosis as the basis for their treatment. Even though rating discomfort and disease in numbers and scales simply does not fit with the convictions held by some naturopathic practitioners, there is public demand for these services and many of them feel pressure to comply. At the same time, using allopathic diagnoses and diagnostic tools does serve two purposes in a naturopathic setting: building a bridge between the practitioner and patient, and making use of what is seen as universal knowledge.

Being on the Same Wavelength

First and foremost, the acceptance and use of laboratory tests can build a bridge between the practitioner and the patient, who is used to communication in allopathic-scientific terms (see also Cassidy 1995, Salkeld 2014). The application and explanation of the tests provide the patient with a feeling of safety and common language, and reassure them that their problems and diseases are understood or, as Smith-Morris puts it, the diagnosis conveys shared meaning (2016). As one practitioner at GNH pointed out:

> For diagnoses we use allopathic words. We cannot rely on Iris diagnoses; they are not competent enough for the patients. If you want to convince the patient, it has to be scientifically-rooted. That's why we have studied both diagnosis systems. And there is no harm in using these methods. What we need is credibility, not only claims, so that everybody is convinced – the media, the other medical systems and the rest of the world. That's why we use methods for diagnosis that everybody understands, and these are allopathic.

The importance of reassuring the patient that the doctors are on the same wavelength gains weight over the duration of treatment: Patients demand assurance and reassurance of the treatment's success. As a consequence of patients' frequent request for evidence of effectiveness, laboratory tests have either become institutionalized within most professional and psycho-nutritional naturopathic hospitals, centers and ashrams, or affiliations have been established with outside laboratories. Tests, scans and screenings are conducted at regular intervals so that patients can visualize their progress.

The Universality of Allopathic Knowledge

A second reason for legitimizing allopathic tests and scans is the fact that these diagnostic methods are not necessarily seen as exclusively allopathic knowledge but rather as universally applicable knowledge. This view is supported by BNYS doctors as well as by other medically-educated clerks. With some exceptions, most Naturopaths (even most psycho-nutritionals) regard scientific subjects like anatomy, biochemistry and organology to be general knowledge with a varying degree of relevance to their own practice. Even those who refuse to carry an officially-acknowledged naturopathic title show interest in measured functions, their occurrence in the body, and the way they are presented by Allopaths and natural scientists. These explanations are not so much seen as an alternative knowledge system that can be translated into "naturopathic terminologies" or integrated into a "naturopathic ideology," but rather they are looked upon with respect and curiosity and considered to be universal knowledge. For most practicing Naturopaths, diagnostics and tests are a way of understanding the body in order to improve treatment, but they are not mandatory.[2]

These two reasons for why the use of allopathic diagnostics in Naturopathy do not contradict each other: First, patients demand a common language and most already bring a fixed diagnosis from Allopathy. In the transcript excerpt above, the first patient arrived at the hospital with the lab results and a diagnosis of chronic tonsil infection. The second patient likewise visited the naturopathic hospital in order to heal a pre-diagnosed ailment, in his case high blood pressure. While patients in naturopathic hospitals sometimes receive a naturopathic etiopathogenetic explanation of their disease, other times they receive a biomedical explanation or even a conglomeration of both paradigms. The first patient's doctor traced the tonsil infection to his use of "unnatural" tooth paste, which is clearly an example of toxification, even if it is a local one (*"it will absorb your enamel, all the calcium, everything from your teeth as well as your jaws"*). However, the Naturopath links the second patient's ailment to his genes (*"his father also has it; its genetic"*) as well as to an organic cause, namely renal failure.

Second, most Naturopaths also rely on the allopathic diagnosis. Most indeed take anatomy and blood tests seriously. For the Naturopath in the transcript, the diagnoses of both patients were "real" and not negotiable. Still, they do not see the point in attempting to prove the success of naturopathic treatment as

---

2 A very small number of Naturopaths, however, deny a subdivision of the body into organs, essentials and liquids, or at least highlight the irrelevance of a science taking care of such matters. Since they are the minority, they are excluded from this argument.

they believe that patients do. Naturopathic treatment is coherent in itself to such an extent that ongoing verification is redundant.[3] The doctor in the transcript emphasized the lab results in order to appear more professional in front of the patient and myself. In her studies of ayurvedic practitioners, Langford (2002) notes a similar gap in the "*awkward disjunctures between a biomedical anatomy and a seemingly mythographic physiology*" (ibid:15). In practice, however, this "*binarism of symptom and disease*" (ibid: 21), as she calls it, is irrelevant in the patients' healing process. This is also the case for naturopathic patients. The allopathic diagnosis is accepted and acted upon. Naturopaths are more concerned with the treatment of the patient than the determination or labeling of the condition. In the case of the first patient, the Naturopath recommends total abstinence from toothpaste and instead prescribes "*herbal paste*" and "*[swishing] a spoonful of cold-pressed organic sesame oil in the mouth.*" The second patient is advised to discontinue his allopathic medication and instead concentrate on gooseberry paste and other elements of the naturopathic diet. There is no alternative than naturopathic treatment for any kind of ailment – it is not used complementarily.

Recording the Diagnosis

The diseases that are recorded in case sheets or statistics therefore refer to the diagnostics obtained from allopathic medicine (or at least the diagnoses that patients are prepared to reveal) or to a vague, perhaps unclassified pain. When a patient arrives at a naturopathic hospital, there is a standardized admission form that is used as the point of reference for the doctors during the treatment.[4] At this point, the naturopathic doctor documents the patient's personal history of illness, family history, treatments taken in the past, current diagnosis, and general lifestyle issues such as the use of alcohol, tea, tobacco or coffee. The questionnaire also inquires about eating habits, stools, sweating, appetite, recreation, bathing and clothes. The focus is clearly on identifying the "errors" in the patient's way of life. These sections are followed by a table to record changes in weight, blood pressure and pulse rate over the course of treatment. The subsequent pages provide space for charts on advised treatment and diet. Those charts are taken to the kitchen staff and treatment assistants, who are

---

3   This is not self-evident. Frank (2004), who conducted a large study on homeopathy in India, pointed out that among his homeopathic practitioners, reassurance is also not a necessary part of their practice. Observing the results and knowing that they work is enough proof of efficacy for the homeopathic practitioners and their patients.

4   Two examples of these admission forms, one from the NLH and one from the MNCC, are presented in the appendix. They are fairly similar and representative of admission forms in naturopathic hospitals.

TABLE 4   *Distribution of diseases in the MNCC*

Obesity	40%
Diabetes	28%
Coronary Artery Disease	16%
Pain	14%
Orthopedic Injury	8%
Miscellaneous	8%
Cancer	5%

Note: Miscellaneous conditions include migraine, hyperactivity, alcoholism, Parkinson's disease, premenstrual syndrome, psoriasis, and elephantiasis. Due to multiple diagnoses in some patients, the percentages total more than 100%.

both responsible for implementing these instructions from the doctors. This admission process indicates that the patients themselves are primarily responsible for labeling their disease. However, many patients decide to bring along their allopathic laboratory test results, which are then attached to the case sheet. Table 4 depicts the most common diagnoses that patients declare during their preliminary consultation at the MNCC hospital. Since long-term statistics are rarely collected, the following percentages represent a snapshot from a sample taken between 21 April – 5 August 2010. The MNCC maintains a record book with basic background data such as patient name, disease and duration of stay. In order to create this figure of the distribution of diseases, I used one record book from the above-mentioned period of time and analyzed almost 500 files. Again, the naming of the disease retained in the book always referred to the diagnosis the patient was given in an allopathic hospital or clinic prior to arriving at the naturopathic hospital.

Since this particular center focuses on fasting, one might assume that this is the reason for the high number of patients reporting problems with obesity. In fact, the distribution of diseases is quite similar to other hospitals visited in this study. The only exception to this is the GNH in Thrissur, which specializes in treatment for renal failure and therefore the majority of patients suffer from kidney disease. The fact that obesity is the most common patient affliction is concordant with the main focus of naturopathic hospitals: A change of diet, whatever it might look like specifically.

Some overweight patients in naturopathic hospitals aim for quick success for a special event, rather than being prepared for a long-term lifestyle change. During my stay in the MNCC there was a group of young patients, both male and female, trying to quickly shed excess weight. Two of them wanted to get married in the near future but believed that they would have a better chance of finding a suitable partner with a slimmer body. Therefore, both stayed in the hospital for more than one month. The girl was forced to do so by her parents, since they had been unsuccessful in finding her a husband because of her weight issues.

The second most common diagnosis is diabetes (mostly Type II diabetes mellitus), an affliction that often goes hand-in-hand with obesity. Together with coronary artery disease (CAD), the third most common diagnosis, this situation reflects the general increase of these afflictions in Kerala (as elucidated in Wilson 2010a, Chacko 2003, Xavier et al. 2008 and Gupta 2005[5]). The fourth most common diagnosis is a symptom complex labeled "pain" that occurs in various parts of the body, often manifesting as frequent headaches, chronic back pain or vague muscle pain. In my sample, patients experiencing pain from an unknown cause had usually not been officially diagnosed beforehand, at least not in a way that was satisfying or helpful for the patient. Indeed, allopathic doctors in general often fail to identify a proper diagnosis for non-specific pain and therefore dismiss these patients' complaints as psycho-somatic. Orthopedic injuries can cause muscle wrenching or sprains after an accident, for example. Naturopathic treatment is generally more affordable than an in-patient rehabilitation program and it includes similar massage and exercise components.

Diagnoses of cancer and non-curable diseases like Parkinson's are rather rare but still exist. Typically in these cases, patients seek naturopathic care to manage the side effects of allopathic therapies.

Naturopathic doctors tend to combine the diseases in the first four groups (obesity, diabetes, CAD, and pain) into a broad category called lifestyle diseases.

---

5   Recent WHO estimates (2015) illustrate the changing landscape of chronic disease in India, and the challenges that face its health care system. The number of overweight males will rise from 22% in 2005 to 31% in 2015, while the number of overweight women will swell from 21% in 2005 to 29% in 2015. The number of people who die from a chronic disease will climb by 18% (see also Gopinath 1997) and the number of diabetes deaths by 35%. Death from infectious diseases, maternal and perinatal conditions and nutritional deficiency combined will also increase by 15%. Osella and Osella (2010) colorfully describe how diet varies in Kerala depending on religion. They note that feasting on vegetarian Hindu *sadhya* provides a rich calorie intake. However, everyday Muslim sociality certainly does not pale in comparison; when people meet, "*food is never too far away*" (ibid: 189). Chubby movie stars like Mohanlal or Mammootty are celebrated. As much as the statement "*you have become a little fat*" might irritate an adult German woman such as myself, that comment by a Malayali is meant as a positive appreciation of one's physique.

They believe that the main cause of these diseases is a lifestyle out of tune with nature. In general, the emphasis is on chronic diseases in most naturopathic hospitals, while acute diseases are rare. This observation is in line with Frank's research on homeopathy in India (2004). He claims that medical division of labor exists among practitioners in India. Acute diseases are treated mainly by Allopathy while patients with chronic diseases turn to other systems such as Ayurveda. Based on results from several studies, Frank further explains that Ayurvedic treatment most commonly deals with skin diseases, sexual troubles, arthritis and paralysis. This trend is also evident in the diagnostic patterns in naturopathic hospitals with the additional component of obesity and long-term diseases such as cancer or Parkinson's disease. Although I did find archived files of patients with acute diseases such as sinusitis or diarrhea who sought treatment in naturopathic hospitals, I did not encounter any such patients during my actual research.

Due to the chronic nature of most diseases in naturopathic hospitals, patients do not seem to expect quick healing, with the exception of a few patients attempting quick weight loss for a special event. In general, the average duration of in-patient hospital treatment is between two and three weeks, which is a significantly longer timeframe than what my participants had previously experienced in other hospitals or medical systems in Kerala. While Connor and Samuel (2001) point out that patients in India have a strong tendency to be impatient and expect results within a few days, naturopathic patients do not seem to be in a hurry.[6]

3   Dodging the Stigma of Mental Illness: A Female Occurrence

Surprisingly, a psychiatric diagnosis is very rare in naturopathic hospitals. In my first encounters with naturopathic practitioners, mainly psycho-nutritionals who were not working regularly in a specific hospital but traveled between

---

6   The average duration of treatment depends on the disease and, of course, on the time a patient wants to spend in the hospital. Some hospitals require a minimum duration of stay and a special program for that period of time – for example, a fixed 3-week program. Obese patients are put on fasts at the beginning of the treatment, which requires several extra days for the body to adjust. Apart from these fixed programs, hospitals and patients decide on an individual basis about the length of the patient's stay. For more severe diseases the hospital generally asks patients to remain a little longer, so that a stay extending over months or even a year is not unheard of in some institutions. In addition, some patients attend the clinics in intervals, staying at home during the intervening period in order to be with their relatives or to return to work.

health camps, I got the impression that the number of reported psychiatric cases was high. This may have been due to my personal interest[7] and to the fact that several patients in the health camps spoke about their mental ailments quite openly. In contrast, a psychiatric diagnosis turned out to be a rare phenomenon during my actual hospital stays.[8] In fact, according to the files in the MNCC, hardly a single case had an official mental illness diagnosis. However, after spending some time getting to know the patients, I discovered that some of them deliberately withheld their history of mental ailments from the hospital staff and other patients for fear of being stigmatized.[9]

According to Kirmayer (1989), a psychiatric diagnosis can be particularly stigmatizing because it possesses an inherent focus on the individual, an emphasis that may be discordant when existing within a less-individualistic cultural context. In order to explain the political and social significance of stigma in Kerala, it is necessary to expand the scope at this point: due to its high prevalence over a range of health issues and its attached social stigma, mental health is a touchy topic in India (see for example Sumeet and Jadhav 2009, Hackett and Hackett 1990, Weiss et al. 2006, Math et al. 2007, Chua 2014). Over the last four decades, policy-makers have attempted to respond to the mental health needs of the population and launched several programs such as the *Mental Health Act* of 1987 (revised in 2002) and more recently the *Mental Health Care Bill* in 2013 (MHCB 2015, Weiss et al. 2001). The shared aim of the different programs is to create and increase awareness about mental health issues, or in other words, to increase mental health literacy. In this understanding, people are regarded as being more literate if they are thoroughly informed about Western biomedical conceptions of disease, where the functioning of genes or biochemistry in the brain is seen to be responsible for both the psychological ailment and the attached stigma (Watters 2010). The expected solution to mental "weakness" or problems is thus seeking help from a psychologist or psychiatrist.

However, this hereditary concept of mental illness can serve to increase social stigma more than diminish it, particularly for women in Kerala. It not

7 I was employed on a project on the conceptualization of depression in different medical systems in Kerala; therefore, anything related to mental health issues was one of my first inquiries when meeting a new practitioner from any kind of medical system or way of treatment.

8 Another reason for the low percentage of psychiatric diseases in naturopathic hospitals might be the fact that this field is well-covered by Allopathy and for the past decade or so also by Ayurveda (Lang and Jansen 2010, 2013).

9 The social negotiation of stigma has already been topic of anthropological research in the 1980s (Good and Good 1986, Good 1994, Young 1981).

only worsens their "bad hand of cards" during marriage negotiations but the larger family appears in a questionable light. Labeling a person as mentally ill can have enormous legal consequences such as divorce (Dhanda 2000), and it can decrease one's social standing and employment opportunities. As a woman in India, it is generally safer to avoid talking too frankly about one's past history with mental illness. Due to the risk of social isolation, for some people it is simply unbearable to admit being treated for psychological problems in any medical system.

Yet, for some of the patients I met, Naturopathy offered a way around this risk. With its promise of holistic treatment and a lifestyle correction, there is no stigma attached to a stay in a naturopathic hospital. Because most naturopathic hospitals simply accept the diagnosis provided by the patient and organize their treatment accordingly, this affords patients the opportunity to alter a diagnosis into a more pleasant or socially-accepted condition. Having an unhealthy lifestyle and experiencing mental health challenges often go hand-in-hand; as such, there is no need for a patient to lie. The cases of Sruthi and Merrin will illustrate this phenomenon.

Sruthi's Story

I met Sruthi, a 26-year old woman, in a psycho-nutritional hospital in Kozhikode. According to her patient file, Sruthi was in the hospital for joint pain. Her wrist problems prevented her from operating a computer keyboard, a necessary task for her job in a call center. She was accompanied by her two-year old daughter and her diabetic mother, who occasionally slept in the hospital and also took part in some of the therapies. Her treatments consisted of early-morning Yoga classes, twice-daily wet bandages and occasional massages for the wrists, a daily spinal bath for relaxation, a twice-daily serving of raw fruits, and a noontime serving of raw vegetables. In the early afternoon, Sruthi took part in lessons on naturopathic lifestyle and spent every evening in the hall receiving meditation lessons.

In the middle of my own three-week hospital stay, Sruthi asked me to take care of her daughter during her spinal bath since her mother was absent. I had already conducted a standard interview with Sruthi before this encounter so I sat down, relaxed on her bed, and arranged toy blocks for her daughter. Through the open bathroom door Sruthi told me how convinced she was by naturopathic treatment, because it *"provides holistic treatment."* *"Finally,"* she added, *"I do not feel any tension anymore."* After a moment of silence, Sruthi began to tell her story. When she was growing up, she said that she always felt a little different, as if she had emotions or tension that other children did not. Once, she fell in love with a boy at school and was convinced that it was her destiny to marry him. She heard voices in the radio confirming her desire to merge spiritually with her teenage classmate. The situation escalated when Sruthi confronted him heatedly in front of her classmates. She received a punishment from the school as well as from her parents for her inappropriate behavior. After that episode, Sruthi increasingly disengaged from social contacts, stopped eating and became very quiet. Her family was worried about her and took her to several allopathic hospitals. Sruthi passed through a complete physical exam and finally ended up seeing a psychiatrist, who diagnosed her with depression and anxiety disorder. Sruthi received medication and frequently visited the psychiatrist's outpatient clinic. When she turned 22 and the family began to search for a decent groom, her parents decided to stop her medication and the visits to the psychiatrist. The plan succeeded, and Sruthi soon married an attractive engineer in a promising position in Dubai.

After she gave birth to her daughter, however, she felt scared, lonely and "*had tension again*." Her situation was revealed when Sruthi escaped from her in-laws' home twice in the middle of the night to return to her parents' home. At that point Sruthi finally confessed her psychiatric history. She explained how scared she was about being thrown out of her in-laws' house and having no home for herself and her daughter. Sruthi's husband was unable to cope with the situation and increasingly treated his wife "roughly" – for example, letting her carry all the heavy bags at the market and scolding her day and night. Her father-in-law decided to send her to a naturopathic hospital; he had been there a number of times for his obesity and saw "*many cured, even mental cases.*" Sruthi took sick leave at the call center due to strong pain in her wrists and sought treatment at the naturopathic hospital. In the admission interview she did not mention any mental health issues and in the almost four weeks she had been there she never told the hospital staff. Sruthi enjoyed the daily routines in the hospital; she liked raw food, the pleasant treatments and, as she emphasized, the Yoga and group mediation relieved the tension she felt. There was no need to explain her reason for the hospital stay other than a lifestyle change to decrease wrist pain. Her in-laws and her own family visited her often in the hospital. She summarized her story with the words, "*Now all the problems are gone; I am very much free now and feeling very good.*"

Sruthi and Sruthi's in-laws aimed to limit the damage of having a "mental case" in the family. If not wrist pain, Sruthi would probably have come up with another similarly socially-acceptable diagnosis or simply voiced the concern to improve her diet. Due to its "open house" policy, a psycho-nutritional hospital offers the possibility to do so. After coming back home from the hospital, Sruthi continued to practice Yoga for the tension she felt and decided to either continue going to the naturopathic hospital once a year or to hire a private Yoga teacher to keep her reminded of the special techniques that were very effective for her. She also liked that she lost weight in the hospital and therefore felt *"fresh and new"* when she left. As she told me in a short follow-up interview in 2012, her in-laws supported her better now.

Merrin's Story

Merrin was 25 when I met her at a professional hospital close to Taliparamba. She had shared a hospital room with her non-English-speaking mother for over a month. Both of them are Christian and had traveled all the way from Varkala. According to her patient file, Merrin was admitted for overweight, while her mother was coping with the symptoms of menopause. Her mother's treatment consisted of three glasses of fresh juice per day as her only food, in addition to water treatments and oil massages. Merrin was put on a radical coconut water fast and also received steam baths and oil massages. Merrin was about to become a biomedical doctor and now wanted to get married. However, it was difficult to find a groom that would accept her overweight so she was trying eagerly to lose weight. In order to make the naturopathic fast more effective, Merrin formed a hiking group together with myself and two other patients, walking twice a day up and down the hills of northern Kerala. During these walks, Merrin talked about some of her mother's problems, until she finally agreed to have a formal interview on this topic. According to Merrin, her mother started having mental problems two years ago following problems with swollen feet, a painful knee, and resulting mobility restrictions. Together with the symptoms of menopause, this caused a strong depression, diagnosed by Merrin:

> M: "She has some problems here" (moving her finger next to her face in a circular motion). "I used to get very irritated by this."
> Me: "So what do you do?"
> M: "I just keep going and don't talk to her. If you go and talk to her she will be like cry, cry, cry. Mainly her problem is anxiety. Even for small things she will get really very tense and anxious. She is not that much of a normal person anymore. If somebody changed their character like she did we would call that a psychiatric problem. I was giving her some medicines for that but nowadays she is not taking all these medicines, because they told her to stop everything here."
> Me: "That means you told the doctors here?"
> M: "She didn't and I didn't because she will say that I am calling her mad. We are not telling anyone." (voice lowers) "Really I can't talk about that. I can't tell what happened to her. I already have enough problems" (pointing to her stomach – referring to her weight).

For Merrin, a common treatment for her and her mother at the same time seemed self-evident. She believed that reducing weight and the calmness of the hospital would improve her mother's condition. Due to the fear that she would not find a husband for herself, Merrin never took her mother to a psychiatric doctor but instead hoped that the self-prescription and the naturopathic treatment would help her sufficiently. However, she did plan to put her mother back on psychotropic medication after they left the naturopathic hospital.

Merrin used the access to medication that she has through her education in order to keep her mother's condition private. The fact that she wanted to lose weight at the same time that her mother's situation deteriorated was a serendipitous coincidence and facilitated their co-habitation in the hospital. There was no need to tell their relatives or employees at the naturopathic hospital about her mother's symptom complexes; all they conveyed during the admission process were the non-mental ailments such as her painful knee and menopausal symptoms. Unfortunately this story did not end so well, and in 2015 when I last spoke with her, Merrin still used most of her energy to care for her mother rather than leading a married life with a reputable husband.

Both stories reveal that naturopathic treatment is used as a loop-hole to avoid stigmatization and its social consequences. It is considered inappropriate to speak openly about mental ailments, particularly for women in Kerala; people might suspect that they will pass the ailment to somebody else. Therefore, the naturopathic hospital gives them the opportunity to offer an alternative diagnosis with no stigma attached. Indeed, "lifestyle correction" is an accepted goal for everyone visiting a naturopathic hospital. This makes Naturopathy an inclusive system of medicine. In the field of mental health care in India, Naturopathy provides autonomy and agency for the patient similar to "folk" mental health care (Quack 2012).

4   Conclusion

In the context of the naturopathic hospital, both patients and physicians not only accept biomedical language but actively make use of it in particular contexts. Biomedical language thereby creates the frame of reference for determining the medical condition of patients, particularly during the admission process. For this, physicians as well as patients employ biomedical terminology for the purpose of labeling. There is an implicit agreement between both actors not to question the allopathic diagnosis that is brought into the hospital from the outside. The actual act of diagnosis is externalized to the allopathic system of medicine. Biomedical language is considered to be universal knowledge and the basis for communication: It becomes common ground.

To evaluate this social fact one has to consider the importance of diagnosis for the naturopathic hospital. While in any allopathic treatment setting the act of attaching a medical label to a patient catalyzes power and agency relationships between all involved actors (physicians, patients, nurses, etc.), in the naturopathic hospital the diagnostic process is reduced to an administrative act in order to complete the file. It is stripped of its medical significance. This becomes particularly obvious during the admission interview: There, patients are asked to enumerate and specify current and former health conditions. Naturopathic practitioners do not question these self-reports. They do not bother convincing patients to have a medical check-up, nor do they conduct it themselves.

Instead, medical priority in naturopathic hospitals is given to therapy. While the extent of treatment individualization varies to some degree between the different hospitals (professional vs. psycho-nutritional), there are several ideological common grounds, such as the high importance given to nutrition, physical exercise and non-substance-based treatment techniques. Even though some professional hospitals aim to provide personal and individual treatment details, to a large extent the patients still consider naturopathic treatment to be homogenous at least in comparison to other medical systems.

The patients' perspectives in this context are most interesting. They strongly believe the naturopathic claim to be a holistic medical system that treats the whole person. Taking this into account, the insignificance of diagnosis provides them with the extra benefit – compared to other medical systems – of receiving medical treatment detached from social implications. They can communicate socially accepted and non-stigmatized diseases to their kin and peers. The knowledge and power to handle their diagnoses lies in their own hands. As the cases of Sruthi and Merrin have demonstrated, this can have very positive effects on some patients' social lives outside the hospital. Both used other diagnoses to get treatment in naturopathic hospitals in order to dodge the stigma of being marked with a personal or family history of mental illness.

Externalizing medical knowledge and practice to the outside of the hospital and even the outside of the medical system provides both physicians and patients in naturopathic hospitals with new agency. The former are able to focus and implement a core ideological concept of the movement, i.e. the equality of people and diseases, as well as providing agency to their patients. The latter have the opportunity to receive naturopathic treatments and lifestyle modifications that are independent of their actual condition. The insignificance of medical diagnosis in the naturopathic treatment context thereby contributes to the creation of the hospital as a social and political site.

CHAPTER 7

The Efforts of Freedom: Patients' Role in Achieving Medical Independence

In seeking health care, patients generally do not differentiate between psycho-nutritionals and professionals, the two groups of Naturopaths. In spite of the professionals' sustained efforts to differentiate themselves from any form of non-college-trained Naturopathy, the type of hospital in which health-seeking patients finally receive treatment is due to other factors. The locality of the hospital and the advice received from their relatives, friends, co-workers or neighbors play a significant role in a patient's selection of hospital. Most prospective patients learn about Naturopathy from other patients. More rarely, media work such as the article below has been successful in attracting some patients: Announcements in newspapers, articles recommending natural diets or self-help columns give the public an initial insight into the theory and practice of Naturopathy[1] (see Figure 10 for an example newspaper article).

Finally, regular health camps organized by various naturopathic groups attract attention in local neighborhoods. In all of these cases, the opportunity to receive a wide variety of treatments at a low cost is alluring.

Patients are rather pragmatic in their help-seeking behavior. Even after being treated for a long period, patients at the NLH do not know that they are being cared for by a practitioner without a medical degree. In cases where they have found out, they do not seem surprised or perturbed. Seeing the many patients who have experienced positive effects from the treatment seems to assure them of having made the right decision. Likewise, patients being treated in professional hospitals do not seem to have preferences regarding the education of Naturopaths. Although some of them find the treatment in professional hospitals fairly complicated and may prefer the simple methods of the psycho-nutritional hospitals, there is no awareness or interest in the rival naturopathic treatment method. I argue that the respective ideological stance enacted by practitioners does not filter down to patients in the intended manner.

The latter statement is the focus of this last chapter. I analyze how the logic of naturopathic therapy in itself prevents patients from fulfilling its idealized aim: to be a once-learned, forever-implemented ideology and related set of treatment applications. By presenting the cases of two core groups of

---

1   Sunday Express Thailand (2008), used here for the non-Malayalam-speaking readership. There are articles in Malayalam newspapers with similar content.

© KONINKLIJKE BRILL NV, LEIDEN, 2016 | DOI 10.1163/9789004325104_010

A natural therapy for children with HIV/Aids is tested at an orphanage in Thailand

By Analaya
SUNDAY XPRESS
Several of the orphans at the Suthatinee Noi-in Foundation's home in Yasothon - are HIV-positive.
To supplement the retroviral drugs they were already taking, in May last year they were introduced to a natural therapy by Jacob Vadakkanchery, a healer

from Kerala in southern India. The foundation spends Bt500,000 a month on drugs to ease the struggle of its HIV-positive children, but there are still several funerals a month. When the doctor first met the children there were four who were so weak that they weren't expected to survive more than a month.

Dr Jacob Vadakkanchery

"This year, to my astonishment no one has died since the introduction of the natural therapy. The children are healthy and happy," claims the healer.

"This shows that there are effective treatments against Aids," says Vadakkanchery, chairman of the Nature Life Hospital in Kerala, whose theory is based on letting the body heal itself.

Along with thousands of patients with various diseases from around the world, the healer says he has also successfully treated some 500 HIV-afflicted patients in India and Cambodia.

Vadakkanchery's philosophy is that drugs can do more damage than good. "Anti-retroviral drugs are more harmful than the disease," is his controversial claim.

He suggests that toxins can be eliminated from the body with a diet of healthful, energising food, mainly fruit and vegetables. Coconut juice is full of nutrients and ideal for healing the body, Vadakkanchery explains.

Interferons are natural proteins produced by the body in its fight against foreign agents such as viruses, parasites and tumour cells. Diet, adds the healer, is the best way to encourage this defence.

"Food is your medicine - your

XTRA

VADAKKANCHERY'S DIETARY CURES

>> **Constipation:** watermelon, papaya, apple, lime juice, ripe banana, orange

>> **Colds:** papaya, pineapple, citrus fruits, carrot, celery, beetroot, ginger, cinnamon, mint

>> **Diabetes:** passion fruit, carrot, celery, bitter gourd

>> **Heart disease:** coconut water, lotus seeds, onion, celery, garlic

>> **Cancer:** grapes, citrus fruits, apple, carrot, asparagus, wheatgrass juice, tomato, broccoli

>> **Dr Jacob**
Vadakkanchery's Thai-language book "Thammachart Bumbud" is available in good bookstores for Bt160. Visit NatureLifeHospital.org for more about his work.

body makes new cells out of food," says Vadakkanchery, who claims to have been disease-free for 28 years.

Other treatments he recommends include yoga, exposure to morning sunlight, water therapy, mud packs and, last but not least, encouragement and support. "With enough of these, a person's chance of survival grows," he says.

FIGURE 10   *Newspaper article promoting naturopathic treatment*

naturopathic patients, I demonstrate the difficulty of being truly empowered by the treatment. The chapter is organized in the following manner: First, I explain the differentiation of patients in naturopathic hospitals in terms of reasons for seeking care. I delineate the following groups: so-called "better off" patients and a contrasting group of patients with "no other option." Secondly, I investigate the concrete obstacles that patients face in embodying naturopathic principles, which are closely connected to the effects of treatment. Altogether, this chapter places the experiences of patients at the forefront and allows their voices to be heard.

1   Medical Biographies in Naturopathic Treatment

This chapter illustrates the background of several exemplar patients, sharing their motivations, hopes and experiences of naturopathic treatment.[2] They

2   There have been several attempts to conceptualize what hospital patients experience during their healing processes with the help of Victor Turner's (1977) theoretical conceptualization

will not be categorized by the hospital they are actually visiting, whether it be psycho-nutritional or professional, but by a different set of criteria. There is no such thing as a typical naturopathic patient. However, certain similarities, tendencies and differences can be identified among people who seek naturopathic expertise.

Of the approximately forty formal interviews and more than two dozen informal talks with patients, two major groups emerged: I call the first group "better off" patients, which is comprised of two subgroups. They are able to afford treatment in other medical systems, particularly allopathic medicine. Some of them, the first subgroup, regard naturopathic treatment as complementary to their usual habit of consulting an allopathic doctor. It is their specific condition of "lifestyle" problems that motivates them to stay in a naturopathic hospital instead, but in general, they are very supportive of allopathic medicine. However, those in the second subgroup of the "better off" patients want to avoid what they regard as invasive allopathic interventions. For them, the healing power of Naturopathy becomes a serious alternative and they are therefore critical of Allopathy.

The second major group, here called "no other option" patients, do not have the economic means to undergo any other form of medical treatment in the region. Due to the low cost of in-patient treatment, patients in this group have no other choice but to stick with Naturopathy. Of course, this model of two main groups does not apply universally to all naturopathic hospital patients; however, it serves to provide a general picture of their orientation, beliefs, and motivations. I will examine these groups in detail below using patient case studies drawn from the categories depicted in Figure 11.

---

of "rites of passage." Rites of passage are part of ritual theories and comprise three stages: (1) the phase of separation, a "dis-integration" of the individual from a former social category; (2) the phase of transition, where the person is in a so-called liminal stage or "betwixt and between"; and (3) the last phase of reintegration into the new category or identity. While models are very rare in anthropology, this one has been embraced and eagerly employed to describe quite a few phenomena typically at the heart of anthropological research: death, marriage, initiations, religious ceremonies, and graduations, to name a few examples. Medical anthropologists such as Agic (2012) and Long et al. (2008) used Turner's concept to describe the stages a patient goes through during medical treatment. I elected not to use this analytical lens because, due to my own "healer-shopping," I was not able to follow a significant number of patients longitudinally.

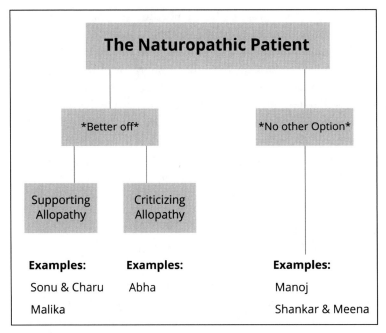

FIGURE 11   *The naturopathic patient*

2   **"Better off" Patients**

When Alter (2004, 2015) talked about naturopathic patients, he was referring to a group of English-educated middle-class patients who wanted to slow down their modern, fast-paced, stressful life in Indian metropolitan areas. Alter found these patients in a naturopathic ashram in the outskirts of Delhi. Their health problems were mainly related to their urban life circumstances and they sought relief in fancy fitness centers, hydrotherapy clinics, and an Ayurvedic Health Club with experts in oil therapy from Kerala.[3]

Middle-class patients can indeed be found in South Indian naturopathic hospitals and ashrams. However, since Kerala is less urbanized due to its lack of international metropolises like Delhi or Mumbai, these patients do not predominate. Naturopathic hospitals in South India do not have the same facilities as the BNCHY described by Alter or the services available in the Jindal Nature

---

3   The relationship between the emerging middle class and changing eating habits is also elucidated in Appadurai 1997, Brosius 2010, Banerji 2010, Beckenridge 1995, Fernandes 2006, Ganguly-Scrase 2009, Liechty 2003, Varma 1998 and Young 1999.

Cure Center in Bangalore.[4] Despite this, depending on the naturopathic institution, middle-class, English-educated patients constitute a significant proportion of the total clientele. At least one Malayali can be found in every hospital who emigrated to the Gulf for either a short- or long-term period, especially in Kerala (see also Osella and Osella 2008, 2000). In addition to that, Malayalis who moved to Mumbai or other large cities return to the countryside and enjoy being treated in coconut-surrounded naturopathic ashrams. Middle-class patients not only come from far-flung places but from the surrounding neighborhoods and towns. Typically they are very well-informed about their disease, the treatment opportunities, and Naturopathy in general even before they take their first step into the hospital.

Sonu & Charus's Story

For example, Sonu and Charu are a married couple in their early fifties from Mumbai. Back in Mumbai they have two adult sons. Both sons are well-educated; one is a software engineer and the other is a pilot at an international airline. Sonu himself works in the management of the same airline. Charu, who stayed home when her children were young, is now working as a secondary schoolteacher of English. Their parents moved to Mumbai from Kozhikode, where both were born; they met through their parents' Kerala network in Mumbai. As they emphasize, their marriage was a love marriage, though their parents were not unhappy about their choice. Almost every year Sonu and Charu return to Kerala to visit their relatives because they still feel a strong connection to the area, and they speak Malayalam with each other as well as with their children. I met them in the NLH hospital in Kozhikode when they decided to spend three weeks as part of their yearly holiday. Sonu is in the initial stage of Type II diabetes and he suffers from high cholesterol. At the moment he is not taking any kind of medication and he wants to avoid having to do so – he regards naturopathic treatment as the first step towards living a healthier life and being cured "naturally" from diabetes and high cholesterol.

---

4   Jindal Nature Cure in Bangalore was founded in 1978, and was therefore one of the very first naturopathic institutes. It is named after one of the Indian naturopathic pioneers. Nowadays it has a large, impressive campus with professionalized courses of education. Due to the high volume of patients, the location has every naturopathic service one can imagine, even a swimming pool. Visitors are not very welcome since it is only open for patients who stay there for a certain amount of time and immerse themselves completely in the naturopathic world. The campus is very close to the city of Bangalore, which is widely known for its "modern lifestyle." Therefore, the percentage of stressed city dwellers, who fit Alter's definition of the average naturopathic patient, dominate. More information on the Jindal Nature Cure can be found at Jindal 2016.

He receives daily enemas and takes regular sun baths to support the dietary treatment. Charu is very eager to lose at least five kilograms; she explains that in contrast to Kerala, the style of dress in Mumbai makes it more difficult to cover an overweight body. In addition to eating only raw food, she receives regular hip baths. They both believe that their health problems are caused by the sedentary nature of their jobs – they spend most of their time sitting and regularly consume high-calorie food. Since they are not accustomed to living a "simple life" as it is exemplified in the NLH, they complain about mosquitoes, uncomfortable beds without mattresses and the lack of hot water in the bathroom. They have less difficulty coping with the heat in their Mumbai home because they have air conditioning in every room. Sonu additionally misses his TV since he wanted to follow cricket, and he is disappointed that he is the only patient in the hospital interested in the Indian team's record. Charu misses chatting with her girlfriends in the afternoons over chocolate cake and coffee.

Although Sonu and Charu have not exactly enjoyed their sojourn in the NLH hospital, they have decided to stay for the whole period of three weeks in order to *"internalize natural life and therefore keep it fresh in mind when we are back,"* as Sonu explains. Both of them came on the advice of an allopathic doctor who recommended a change in diet, but they had difficulties doing so in Mumbai. A friend of Sonu's parents who lived in the NLH neighborhood told them about the hospital, which they deemed a place without temptation and hence the best location to implement their resolutions. They had planned to consult their allopathic doctor again for a retest after their treatment and should a deterioration of their health emerge, Sonu would seriously consider going on allopathic medication.

Malika's Story

Malika is a 60-year old woman from Chennai whom I met in UGLA in Sivasailam. She stays there for ten days every year in order to lose weight and because she likes the atmosphere of the ashram. She says that it makes her calm after a year of rushing through life, and she considers it to be her personal retreat. She loves sitting on the little swing in the shade of the huge trees, letting her mind wander. Although she enjoys her lifestyle in Chennai, which is characterized by dinners, invitations from friends, and shopping, she feels that a "time-out" is urgently needed once a year.

Just after Malika got married, she had two heart operations and now lives with an artificial wall in her heart. Since then, she has had to take allopathic medication to thin her blood and take care of her diet by avoiding salt and spices. She has become accustomed to her special condition and is still able to travel long distances and enjoy life. She visits her daughter in New Jersey, USA every year for 2-3 months and while there she prefers to wear fancy clothes such as jeans. Therefore she visits the UGLA right before she goes to New Jersey. Her own family and her husband are originally from Andrah Pradesh, but moved to Chennai because they wanted a higher standard of education for their two children. Her husband is a civil engineer and the vice president of a large company and is able to offer her a comfortable life. According to Malika, food plays a special role: She has hired three cooks in order to have a diversity of food. She usually enjoys an Indian breakfast, an Italian lunch and a light continental dinner. Five members of her family have visited UGLA for different ailments such as hypertension or hemorrhoids, and each time the treatment was a great success. Malika lives in the only air-conditioned room in the ashram, although it is December and the thermometer hardly rises above 25 degree Celsius. Aside from her daily visits to the swing, she hardly leaves her room to intermingle with other patients because she does not like *"the male domination in the countryside."* In addition, hygiene is a general concern of hers and she feels that some of them are not particularly clean. She criticizes the hygienic standards of the ashram's cleaning woman, even complaining to the wife of the chief physician, who has become a good friend over the years. Malika really enjoys the treatment, which in her case consists of steam baths and oil massages apart from the very reduced weight-loss diet. She is also convinced that her stays in the UGLA prevent serious diseases in the long-term, believing that periodically cleansing the body can only have a positive effect on her general health.

Similar to Sonu and Charu, Malika does not consider naturopathic measures to be strictly necessary medical treatments. She admits that every year she hopes her stay in the ashram will be a prelude to a life with more raw food and less oil but in the end losing five kilograms and *"relaxing the mind"* once a year is enough success for her. After all her experience with allopathic surgery, she has a lot of respect for the knowledge of those doctors and would not consult a naturopathic doctor for her heart problems.

Like Sonu, Charu and Malika, the patients of this group see Naturopathy as a complementary medicine more than an alternative system. They are not aware of the political connotation Naturopathy carries for many of the practitioners. They consider their stay more like a treatment at a health resort than a hospital. However, there is another subgroup of middle-class patients undergoing naturopathic treatment. This group consists of individuals who seek treatment for life-threatening diseases because they do not like the way that allopathic medication and surgery have handled their disease, and they do not believe in the results of allopathic treatment. They are typically the best-informed patients and have been through a variety of invasive allopathic

interventions such as operations, dialysis, organ transplantation and chemotherapy, which have been traumatizing for some. For these patients, it is not a
question of money but a conviction to stop being helpless and to empower
oneself. At a certain point, they made a decision to regain their agency and to
start collecting information about the possibilities offered by an alternative
medical system. In general, Naturopathy sounded like the least invasive and
most promising option.

Abha's Story

I met Abha in the GNH in Thrissur, where she was undergoing treatment for
chronic renal failure. Originally from Kerala, Abha is a housewife who moved
to Chennai with her husband about three decades ago. Since her siblings and
their children still live in Kerala not far from Thrissur, she decided to undergo
treatment nearby. Her sister searched the Internet and discovered the renal
failure treatment offered at the GNH. Her husband works as a controller in car
manufacturing in Chennai and therefore is not able to visit her often. Abha is
63 years old and has two children. Her daughter studied biology in the USA and
currently lives in Italy with her husband and two children. Abha's son is in his
early thirties and mentally challenged; as such, he is in need of special attention and 24-hour care. In 1977, after her marriage, Abha went to England to
obtain a degree in literature. She speaks English fluently and became my main
source of information in the GNH; she interviewed other patients for me and
was eager to translate the details of her treatment. As she said, she was very
happy to do so since she was "*bored to death*" in the hospital. Before her diagnosis was clear, she underwent more than a year of discomfort, nausea,
vomiting and swollen legs. She sought both allopathic and ayurvedic treatment but received medication for one symptom only, the nausea. Her condition
became worse and she lost an increasing amount of weight. It was only when
she got a complete exam at an allopathic diagnostic center that her renal problems were discovered. After Abha received her diagnosis, she decided to
undergo the obligatory treatment, according to her allopathic doctors: Regular
dialysis to clean the blood, which her body was not able to do itself.

At the age of 63 she could not expect to be at the top of the list for transplantation; in addition, she was not even sure that she wanted a transplant, so she
never even tried to get on the list. Instead, she collected all possible information and reserved a bed in Alma's Hospital in Thrissur. However, when she
arrived for her first pre-check and the dialysis methods were explained to her,
she suddenly found it very cruel and invasive. In the preparation phase she did
not like the idea of "*having chemicals injected*." Nevertheless she was very inse-
cure about alternatives and decided to let surgeons implant the dialysis aditus

in the crook of her arm. At the last moment, however, she revised her decision and followed her sister's advice to be admitted to the GNH. She was scared and felt helpless being tied to a machine, explaining: *"During the treatment you do not have anyone to rely on. You are alone. All your blood will be drained off going through the machine."* When I met Abha, she had already been in the hospital for three months and continued to stay for another three. Apart from special food preparation, Abha received hydrotherapy and sun baths for her swollen legs. When I returned to the hospital nine months later, Abha had been read-mitted. Since we are in frequent email contact, I am aware that Abha is still going back and forth to the hospital for treatment.

For Abha, the only chance to live without dialysis and constant allopathic medication is in the naturopathic hospital. Although her creatine levels con-stantly fell, Abha knew that she had to stick to the naturopathic diet to keep her kidneys working. Her motivations do not constitute a general criticism of allopathic medicine, only some of its practices. She has no intention of freeing Indian society from post-colonial structures by intentionally choosing this sys-tem of medicine. Rather, she feels overwhelmed in the sense that allopathic practices such as dialysis or even surgery are overbearing and invasive towards her body. She does not like the idea of having needles inserted in her skin, or surgeons cutting and operating in her chest. This strong dislike does not extend to oral medication because the act of taking it is connected to the movement of swallowing, which is already familiar to her. Similarly, she is not scared of chemical reactions in her body, but instead sees them as necessary. She sum-marizes her preference: *"I am personally accepting this Naturopathy after avoiding all other systems."*

Additional examples can be found in the rare cancer cases.[5] Most of them do not feel hopeless when they enter naturopathic hospitals, as naturopathic doctors such as Jacob Vadakkanchery affirm, but rather they believe in alterna-tive treatment of their disease. Halliburton (2003) worked with patients who had undergone ayurvedic and allopathic treatment for psychiatric disease and emphasized the importance of a pleasant treatment experience. According to him, patients with severe diseases and without strong time pressure prefer a pleasant therapy within an aesthetic environment. Abha is a typical example of a patient selecting Naturopathy due to its less invasive practices and more convenient and enjoyable applications.

---

5   I only had the chance to conduct short interviews with two cancer patients who were able to afford other treatments such as chemotherapy but refused to do so, since they found this treatment very cruel and were scared of not surviving it.

To conclude, there are two types of "better off" patients who are able to afford allopathic treatment but instead seek naturopathic treatment: the first group resembles Alter's (2004) middle-class definition of patients who visit naturopathic hospitals in order to improve their lifestyle and avoid allopathic medication. However, if these patients had anything "more serious," they would not turn to Naturopathy. Representing the second group, Abha and many other "serious" cases decided to seek naturopathic treatment because they found allopathic treatment or parts of allopathic practices invasive and cruel. Most of them had tried other possibilities such as Ayurveda before, but were not successful. Their critique of allopathic methods is due to personal taste and not to be misconstrued as a general critique of neo-colonial politics.

3   "No Other Option" Patients

In the next part I describe a category of patients who seek naturopathic treatment for financial reasons. They constitute at least half of the patients in naturopathic hospitals and more than two-thirds at the GNH in particular. Their main motivation for seeking naturopathic care is its cost-effectiveness; it is less expensive than any other kind of treatment, including Ayurveda. Although the cost of allopathic medication is far from reaching high-priced Western standards, many Indians cannot afford its long-term use. Medical insurance is hardly affordable, and for a vast majority surgery is a sheer impossibility because of limited financial means (Wilson 2010b). All of my interviewees in this group had previously been in allopathic treatment until it became unaffordable.

Manoj's Story

Manoj had already been at the GNC in Thrissur for over a month when I met him. He shared his room with his wife and his daughter Angelica, a cute seven-year old girl. Manoj and his wife speak very little English, only enough to collect some basic information. After a week, I asked Abha to come to the third floor and help me with the conversation. Manoj's chronic renal failure was discovered five years ago. As he explained, it was caused by Type I diabetes, which he has suffered from since he was a child. He started to feel weak and lost more and more weight until he went for a check-up in his hometown, an area at the edge of Thrissur. His blood counts gave cause for serious concern and Manoj, then working in his uncle's small kiosk, sought treatment at an allopathic hospital in Thrissur. There he was registered for immediate dialysis and put on a waiting list for a kidney transplant. As Manoj is only 33 years old, he would have been taken into serious consideration for the next matching kidney. Manoj and his wife then started collecting money from his family and friends to pay the average dialysis cost of 25,000 rupees per month, until it was his turn for the transplant. With the help of a bank loan and the sale of his brother's car, Manoj was able to undergo dialysis for five months while his wife helped in the kiosk. After five months, however, Manoj and his family ran out of financial resources and had nobody else to borrow money from. Manoj has a very rare blood type and no kidney became available during that time. Through Internet research, Manoj read about the GNH and its renal specialization. He took his wife and daughter and decided to stay for an unspecified period of time. The total amount he spends in the GNH of 2,000 rupees per month is much more affordable than dialysis. Although at this point Manoj cannot afford the total cost of USD $15,000 for a transplant, he is still hoping for a kidney donor. He is quite content with the treatment in the hospital and says:

> See, I have tried this and I am 80 percent satisfied with it. Anyway, it is a state of mind how you react with it, how you get along with these medi-cines [referring to herbal mixtures], and the food. If the body accepts it, it works. I am 80 percent satisfied with it. Twenty percent not, because I know it is not curable. Even Naturopathy cannot cure it, only a trans-plantation can.

The main reason why Manoj stays in the hospital is the affordability of the treatment. Although his renal failure will not be completely cured by Naturopathy, Manoj is able to buy time in the naturopathic hospital without the great expense of allopathic dialysis. He uses this time to wait for a donation from one of his distant relatives or to come up with another financial plan for his transplant. However, he is still paying a heavy price for this decision: He had to disconnect from his life and stay in the hospital full-time. Additionally, his daughter is not able to attend her regular school, since his wife refused to leave her with relatives during their stay in the hospital. Manoj and his family live on the upper floor of the hospital and hardly ever leave their room – he feels too weak to walk up and down the stairs to talk to other patients or go shopping. Most of the time, the young couple stays in the room with their door open, looking after their daughter while she sits in the hall, watching cartoons or playing with other patients.

Shankar & Meena's Story
Shankar and Meena are a retired couple in their late 60s, staying in the GNH at the same time as Manoj. Although they have also been there for over a month

they have never met each other, since Shankar and Meena reside on the ground floor and do not see the point in moving around the hospital. Shankar was a police officer in a small village in Malappuram District and Meena worked as a farmer and cared for the household and their five children. I was introduced to Meena through Abha, who had become friends with her before I arrived at the GNH. Neither she nor her husband speaks any English. Therefore our interviews did not have a formal tone; with Abha serving as translator and explanatory mediator, my casual conversations with Meena enabled the reconstruction of the couple's medical biographies. Only on one occasion did Shankar join our conversation about his medical state, although even then he did not show much interest. Their stay in the GNH was a consequence of his life-long alcoholism: Shankar's liver was seriously damaged – Meena even spoke of early cirrhosis of his liver – and he suffered from emerging dementia, with symptoms of disorientation and short-term memory dysfunction. The couple is unable to live from Shankar's pension alone; therefore, Meena still has to work in the fields.

About three years ago, both of them went to an allopathic doctor who recommended that Shankar completely abstain from alcohol in order to give him at least ten more years of life, but he did not succeed in remaining abstinent. They could not afford to send him to an addiction treatment center where he would be monitored day-and-night and therefore remain safe from the temptation of joining his friends for drinks next to the liquor store. It took three more years and more alarming diagnostic findings before he decided to follow the advice of a friend and gain admission to the GNH. Here the food contributes to the recovery of Shankar's liver, or at least does not make it worse. Shankar does not have the opportunity to leave the hospital, and is thus far away from temptation. Meena hopes that after their stay, which is planned for two or three months, Shankar will completely abstain from alcohol. She already has the feeling that his concentration and short-term memory have improved significantly. Officially he was admitted for his liver problem, but Meena constantly expressed her happiness at the full-time monitoring that forces him to stay sober. As Abha patiently translated: "*Meena thinks there is no other option for him to survive.*" The treatment itself is tailored especially for his liver dysfunction, according to Meena: He receives hot and cold fomentations daily, and twice-daily hip baths and hot foot baths.

Shankar, Manoj and many other poor patients suffering from a variety of diseases such as diabetes, skin problems and even cancer, turn to Naturopathy because the treatment is so affordable. The other options that they investigated were far above their budget. At the GNH, they were able to live in the cheapest way possible and although neither Manoj, Shankar nor Meena really expected a cure, they could at least spend time there while searching for other options. Due to language difficulties, patients with limited English skills are underrepresented in my interviews. Nevertheless, low-caste and/or lower-income people who are simply unable to afford other kinds of treatment constitute a high percentage of patients in naturopathic hospitals and should be studied in more detail.

In terms of health-seeking behavior, the decision of patients to turn to Naturopathy depends on explanatory models of health only in specific cases. Patients such as Sonu, Charu and Malika do indeed believe that their general health problems can be traced back to their lifestyles. They agree that it is primarily their unhealthy or unnatural eating habits that have caused their bodies to become sick. In these cases, Naturopathy is supposed to help them change their eating habits. Therefore, only the patients who are able to afford treatment in other medical systems and do not suffer from an acute, life-threatening disease have explanatory models of health and the body that are analogous to those espoused by Naturopathy. All others seek naturopathic treatment for pragmatic and logistical reasons: Either the hospital is close to their residence or Naturopathy is simply the only option due to its low financial demands.

4   Going On and Off Treatment

As reflected in the cases of Malika, Abha, Sonu, Charu, and Manoj, most patients repeat their naturopathic hospital stays. When I met these patients, all of them were either undergoing a repeat visit or planned to return again in the future.

According to Gandhi's idea of self-sufficient treatment – or as Alter (2004) puts it, the anti-clinic – and the ideology of Dr. Vadakkanchery, patients are only supposed to learn Naturopathic treatment once. At that point, they should understand the basic principles and be ready to apply this knowledge for a lifetime. However, in South India this is not the case; naturopathic patients are much more likely to return to their respective hospitals, sometimes more than once.

There are several reasons for this pattern. Although many patients attempt to change their lifestyle at home in accordance with naturopathic principles, they are confronted with three obstacles to applying their acquired knowledge of naturopathic treatment: First, the social embeddedness of food and the difficulty of integrating naturopathic nutrition into existing customs; second, the challenge of following applied substance-based treatments at home; and third, the impossibility of healing a chronic disease in a short time.

The first and main obstacle is the lack of flexibility in patients' social surroundings. In Kerala, food is embedded in social settings and relationships, and its rejection would be socially unacceptable, whether it be the women cooking lunch for the whole family, the young married couple on a visit to their in-laws, or an older man inviting a friend to watch a cricket game. All of these situations are closely linked with the consumption of food, either snacks or full meals.

Malika, Charu and Sonu are not in constant need of medical care; they are admitted as in-patients in order to increase their general well-being and attractiveness and at the same time ameliorate minor emerging diseases. For Malika, staying at the UGLA is a successful way to stay in shape and regulate her diet. Since Malika calls herself a real gourmet who is interested in *"the whole variety of food [that] earth is able to present,"* and who has the financial means to employ several cooks, staying on a strict diet at home is not possible for reasons of prestige and status. So, she returns to the UGLA every year. Back in Chennai, she is involved in various social activities that are associated with food consumption, hindering her ability to maintain a special diet.

When I met Charu and Sonu they were undergoing naturopathic treatment for the first time; they were, however, already planning to come back after one year in Mumbai. Sonu's diabetes began deteriorating a little while after leaving the NLH. His doctor recommended that he either return to a naturopathic institution or start allopathic medication. Charu similarly regained her weight. Both of them feel that living in a naturopathic hospital like NLH is a fast and easy way to cure their *"lifestyle diseases."* Back in Mumbai with their children and friends, they restarted their *"old lives,"* although they did try to adapt and integrate some of the positive features from the NLH hospital. Sonu decided to eat fruit at least for breakfast and to have a light dinner. It was impossible for him to maintain a naturopathic diet at his workplace, which is the reason why he wanted to concentrate on breakfast and dinner.

An additional factor to the problematic of food's social function is the extraordinary effort that nutritional treatment requires. Even if the patient is willing to risk social exclusion in settings where food plays a major cultural role, he or she experiences difficulties in attempting to live in the same manner as in naturopathic hospitals. The example of the GNH practices is most striking because even for Abha, who has spent months in the hospital and is willing to learn self-treatment, the nutritional advice of the practitioners still seems vague and difficult to repeat. Even on the other end of the naturopathic spectrum, at the hospitals of the NLH, imitating the lifestyle is not as easy as it first appears. One requires constant access to fresh fruits and vegetables, which are limited due to time and money. For example, after a few weeks Charu found it far too exhausting to buy and cut fruits for Sonu every morning in addition to the family's normal breakfast. This entailed pushing back her normal wake-up time to 5:15 AM, which was simply unbearable for her. Herbal mixtures are not necessarily easy to prepare when living in a city or even in another area with slightly different cultivation. Preparing these mixtures requires a lot of time, especially when only a small portion is made fresh every day. Quite a number of patients told me that rice and vegetables are simply cheaper than fruit. When they are in a hurry or only have a short break for lunch, it is easier and more convenient to go to a hotel for meals than to a fruit stand to prepare a naturopathic meal.

For Abha and Manoj in particular, the specific nature of the treatment renders it just too complicated to be managed at home. In the GNH, they pass through a well-organized routine related to the preparation and consumption of food that is difficult for patients to fully comprehend. In addition to food, they receive a mixture of medicinal herbs three times a day. Often they are supposed to be collected locally just two hours in advance of ingestion and then ground manually with a wooden rolling pin. For patients, this procedure is difficult to replicate since most are not from the same locality as the GNH and are unsure whether the same plants grow in their area. In addition to the herbal pastes applied three times a day, the regular meals of breakfast, lunch and dinner all require special preparations. The GNH kitchen staff has a special way of preparing *chapatis*, *putu* and other typical South Indian foods without oil, salt or white flour. The curries, consisting of vegetables such as beetroot and carrots, are prepared in a very particular manner in order to avoid harmful ingredients and formulations.

Eager to return home, Abha tried desperately to understand the nutritional concepts. She spent a lot of time in the GNH kitchen, asking about ingredients and recipes and recording her detailed findings in a notebook. When she returned home in between the first two treatment sessions, her husband hired a household helper. Abha spent many hours teaching her the correct preparation of the herbal mixtures but failed to provide the herbs out of her garden and immediate surroundings. In the end, despite all the effort she made, her creatine level rose again and she decided to go back into the hospital. Here Abha explains her difficulties with naturopathic treatment at home:

> These herbs I have not noticed before,[6] if I take them for a long time I feel released. It is difficult to find them; you have to prepare medicine as paste

---

6   She means that she has not noticed that they are local plants and that they might have a
    medical purpose.

three times a day and the food you have to prepare in the same manner. *Cherula* and *karuka* I can find in the garden in my house but *njerinil* I have not seen. My mother's house where I stay right now is in a small village; there is only one well. It is not in a town area like here. Here you can get more things. But I said I will [go to] the trouble if it reduces my creatine. Then you have no snack at home, no tea, no coffee, not even in the morning, but everybody else is having it. I used to bake cakes but now I cannot have it. No sugar. My husband doesn't like it. Also he doesn't want me to steam and boil vegetables; he said there is no taste. We have to use at least a little oil to fry garlic and onions. When I left the hospital, they gave me a long list but it was not that simple to follow the strict regimen.

Manoj did not even try to learn the specific composition of the herbal mixtures he is taking three times a day. Although he wants to stick to the diet, he sees a lot of difficulties in it:

> The problem is you have to maintain the diet. Normally I prefer anything else, but now I can't go for it; I have to maintain the veg diet, complete veg with no use of oil or fatty things. How can you cook without any oil?

Manoj is convinced that it would be too great a burden on his wife to expect her to learn the recipes. Thus, for Abha and Manoj, staying as an in-patient in the GNH offers the only possibility to extend their lives without worrying about accommodation or undergoing the allopathic methods of treating their disease.

The second obstacle mentioned by patients is the difficulty of undertaking applied treatment at home. A bathtub is needed for most hydrotherapeutic treatments. Since bathtubs are not likely to be found in Indian households, one has the expense of buying one from the hospital and the additional effort of transporting it home. In most of the naturopathic hospitals, special bathtubs for hip baths or arm baths are available to purchase or at least to order. For mud packs one has to collect mud and spread it on a cloth before applying it, which generates considerable cleaning expenses. In Manoj's opinion, he would fail to correctly replicate the applied treatment even if he tried – first, because of the lack of bathtubs in his house, and second, he is convinced that he would not have the time to think about hydrotherapy as soon as he is once again enmeshed in his normal routine. Abha only managed to have her sun baths at home for a couple of minutes twice a day.

Applied substance-related methods need to be organized at home and used a couple of times per day. However, they are not seen as the foundation of naturopathic treatment at home either by practitioners or by patients. Practitioners emphasized that living with the respective foods and without any additional toxins would be enough for a slow cure at home. During my research in South India I only met one person, a young kidney patient from Allapuzha, who bothered to order a bathtub for home treatment; he had had a very positive experience with it.

The third reason for the repetitive nature of hospital visits lies in the nature of the diseases that are prevalent in naturopathic hospitals. Patients seek out Naturopathy mostly for chronic diseases, which cannot be cured quickly but need a longer, consistent treatment period according to both naturopathic and allopathic principles. Obesity, Type II diabetes, and coronary artery disease cannot be healed in three weeks' time. Since most of the patients have daily commitments, it is a common phenomenon to visit the Naturopathy hospitals for a week or two, return home for several months and then return to the hospital for a refresher of the treatment and the respective knowledge. As Abha points out:

> In my understanding if you have a kidney failure, you can have dialysis. Dialysis is a very fast cleaner of the blood. And Naturopathy may be a slow cleaner, you know, maybe less dangerous and less harmful. And when you start living normally it will come up again. This is why I always have to come back.

These three obstacles to home treatment are the main reasons that treatment repetition is characteristic of Naturopathy. In practice, structuring the day according to "natural principles" often limits people's ability to follow their daily life routines, unless one is retired or living alone, or the whole family – if not the community – is taking part in the "project."

5   "My Peace is So Wonderful"

When I started to present at conferences and to engage in personal conversations with anthropologists and non-anthropologists about my research topic, I was usually bombarded with questions from my audience. These questions were typically related to specific treatment methods, the theoretical background of naturopathic concepts, or similarities to German Naturopathy. There was always one person who would ask me skeptically: "*but now, seriously,*

does Naturopathy really work?" It seemed that this was the answer that everybody was waiting for throughout the conversations or presentations. At the
beginning of these interactions and at the start of my research, I repeatedly
explained why anthropologists cannot simply answer this question. It always
depends on the context – it depends on who is receiving treatment for what
kind of disease, in what context, and what that individual understands by
whether a treatment is "working." Since these explanations were rather vague
and therefore disappointing for my audience, I decided to let the patients
speak instead. The following explanations are the answers given by patients
when asked about the efficacy of Naturopathy.[7]

In general, all patients reported strong changes in their body after being in
naturopathic treatment for a while. Due to complete abstention from fat, sugar
and salt, of course, the most striking and visible effect for all patients was a
significant loss of weight. Weight is measured in some naturopathic hospitals
at least once or twice daily to observe a patient's progress. *"Nowadays almost all
patients are eating too much in Kerala and need to lose weight,"* as one doctor
from the MNCC points out. He adds that *"the loss of weight is a first step into
a natural and healthy lifestyle, independent of the disease."* Patients who are
able to afford other treatments and are under naturopathic treatment for lifestyle issues very much appreciate this fast method of weight reduction.
Additionally, many patients told me that their stay in a naturopathic hospital
somehow sharpened their senses. Suddenly, they could taste and enjoy the
sweetness of a papaya, a fruit that is often ignored by Malayalis due to its ubiq-
uitous nature.

Although it is mainly these kinds of patients who experienced initial difficulties adjusting to the food and a life organized around treatments, completely
detached from their normal family and working routine, they ultimately
enjoyed the atmosphere. Since everybody is served the same or similar foods,
the risk of temptation decreases significantly. If naturopathic hospitals did not
exist, Charu and Sonu for example would not be hospitalized at all. Being hospitalized in a naturopathic hospital is therefore a great advantage for them, as
they both agree. Through the afternoon lessons at the NLH, both were eager to
learn exactly what a life in tune with nature would mean.

For patients who would otherwise be hospitalized elsewhere, such as Abha,
Manoj or Shankar, being in a naturopathic hospital has a different meaning.
They do not need to lose weight, but rather they need to decrease the toxins

---

7 Given that this book is not an attempt to write an objective study on the efficacy of Naturopathy,
   the following statements refer to what patients answered to the questions *"Is it working?"* and
   "What is the effect of the treatment on you?"

that their organs cannot metabolize or expel on their own. This effect might sound simplistic, but it is continually proven to the patients by hemograms. Accordingly, these patients can abstain from more invasive allopathic interventions. Manoj expresses his feelings towards naturopathic treatment as follows:

> Naturopathy is nothing but a state of mind. If you are ready to accept this food then suddenly you are free. You do not need any medication anymore. Some people accept it more than others; for some it is really difficult. For me, I am happy here; my peace is so wonderful. I can be without tablets and without anything.

From an impartial point of view, the independence described by Manoj is not maintainable because he has to remain in the hospital and follow the diet fulltime in order to feel free. For him, though, it is obviously the best option. Shankar offers the following statement:

> I am fasting. I thought I could never do this. Normally I have three meals a day, rice, *chapatis*, and at night I have liquor. Here there is nothing like that.[8] After some time I am very comfortable with this diet, with the lifestyle; I feel very happy and comfortable. I don't feel the urge to drink liquor and eat rice.

The feeling of being "released" is frequently described by naturopathic patients – not only the ones who suffer from an addiction problem but also from patients who feel that the *"weight of civilization is taken from me,"*[9] and they do not have to make the financial and logistical efforts to supply themselves with medication on a regular basis. However, as the passive construction of the phrase already indicates, the price of that release is an enforced, extended stay in the hospital. Without the doctor, patients do not have the knowledge or agency to continue naturopathic treatment. They remain docile and dependent upon the naturopathic clinic.

Of course, not all patients in naturopathic hospitals express such positive sentiments about their treatment results. Some patients are never able to deal

---

8   Although he was not fasting in the sense that he was only existing on water or juice, Shankar still experienced the change in diet as fasting. The *chapatis* served in the GNH were not "real" for him, since they were not served with oily or spicy curries.

9   This was a comment by Abha that summarized what Malayalam-speaking patients told her in the clinic regarding how they felt about the effect of naturopathic treatment.

with the lifestyle in naturopathic clinics, and they typically leave the hospital within a few days. Long-term residents also express criticisms, generally relating to the details of treatment. For example, a young obese girl continued to express her disapproval of the ban on fish consumption. She wholly agreed with the raw food policy, enjoyed her Yoga and meditation lessons, and once formulated her new status as *"I know now how I should live; I am feeling good and no urge to have rich cake."* However, in her opinion, Naturopathy needs to be modified to introduce fish to the diet, since *"people are made to eat fish, otherwise they cannot digest."* Similar to the remarks of this young girl, other patients also have ideas about how to increase the efficacy of Naturopathy. When I was in the NLH, there were detailed discussions about the use and necessity of nutritional supplements. Some patients were convinced that taking additional vitamins would increase the efficacy of Naturopathy. As one might imagine, Jacob Vadakkanchery disagreed with this idea.

Thus, patients do not completely agree on Naturopathy's efficacy; instead, there is a continuous discourse on specific details of the diet and applied substance-based treatments and their mechanisms of impact. However, all the patients I interviewed agreed that they felt relaxed, comfortable and even free from their social and addiction-driven compulsions to consume unhealthy food. Even if many of them did not get "cured" during the time that I was acquainted with them, their general attitude towards health, disease and their body changed. For some, if nothing else, Naturopathy provided a feeling of living a life without disease.

6   Conclusion

Patients primarily turn to Naturopathy for the treatment of chronic ailments that have not been successfully cured in other medical systems. Similar to treatment assistants, patients are generally not aware of the political implications of the psycho-nutritional movement. They do not, as a whole, detect nuances or distinctions within Naturopathy as a medical system and therefore regard naturopathic hospitals equally. Instead, they seek treatment at these institutions for two very different reasons: the first group, the financially "better off" patients, aim for a lifestyle change to address their ailments. These patients are represented through the stories of Sonu, Charu and Malika, who all aimed to lose weight and live healthier. They believe in Naturopathy being a gentle method, and hope that it can be easily incorporated into their everyday lives. Only a very small subgroup of these patients is fundamentally critical towards allopathic methods and therefore chooses Naturopathy as an alternative, versus complementary, treatment. These patients are represented through Abha, who wants to avoid dialysis or a transplant for her chronic renal failure.

On the other hand, patients with "no other option" seek naturopathic treatment because it is financially the only way to receive some sort of medical care and to avoid medication or surgery. Here these patients are represented through Manoj, who cannot afford dialysis as he waits for a kidney transplant, and Shankar and Meena, who both aim to keep Shankar away from liquor but are unable to afford the cost of an allopathically-oriented addiction clinic.

Both of these groups are disappointed when they return home, as they find that they are unable to implement their treatment long-term, mostly because the sharing of food is an essential aspect of sociality in South India. This prompts many naturopathic patients to return to the hospital again after unsuccessful efforts at home treatment. Despite this, independent of their disease or actual chances of cure, most patients enjoy their stay in naturopathic hospitals and feel intense, significant, and positive changes in their bodies.

The naturopathic promise is the increased level of patients' agency. "*Come a patient, return a doctor*" is the mantra of Dr. Vadakkanchery and other Naturopaths. However, if one looks beyond the propaganda, it is apparent that the promise of patient empowerment is not realized, either inside the hospitals or beyond. This is true for both types of naturopathic hospitals – the professionals as well as the psycho-nutritionals. Most patients consider naturopathic treatment to be insufficiently transparent, too intricate and, importantly, too anti-social to be sustainable in their daily routines either temporarily or permanently. While the dissemination of the principles underlying Naturopathy are intended to provide people with the means to take control over the treatment of their own bodies, it is actually the naturopathic healer who holds the knowledge and therefore the power during and after medical treatment. This becomes most obvious in the repeated cycles of patients' admission and discharge. The hospital constitutes the very site at which the exceptional medical treatment is performed, yet it is disconnected from people's daily lives and routines. Thereby it becomes a naturopathic space and does not significantly differ from the allopathic hospital despite the idealism of naturopathic ideology.

CHAPTER 8

Conclusion

Naturopathy in South India has increased in popularity in recent years even though it evolved as a medico-political system over the course of two centuries and across several continents. Worldwide it has always been a bottom-up response to social, economic and political changes in society. In India, Naturopathy has provided an ideology of resistance offering munitions in diverse struggles for power. Nutrition is central to the movement not only as a way to maintain health, but also as a political statement. As the analysis throughout this book shows, contemporary South Indian Naturopathy has two main lines of conflict: (1) the ideological line of conflict, and (2) the line of conflict concerning the structural pluralism of Naturopathy. At the same time, there is significant common ground in the implementation of naturopathic treatment.

Lines of Conflict

During late colonialism, Naturopathy was brought to India and contextualized as an alternative form of medical treatment. To counter the biopower of the British empire, Indian naturopathic pioneers made use of treatments created primarily by German anti-modernization medical activists. The former framed and legitimized Naturopathy by adding elements of Indian philosophy such as Yoga, meditation and *panchabutha* elementary concepts. They thereby not only nationalized the phenomenon but also naturalized it: Naturopathy began to appear as natural to Indian patients as other medical systems supported by the British. The result of this historical trajectory is a coherent, self-contained medical system with its own etiopathogenesis and catalog of treatments separate from other accepted medical systems such as Allopathy, Ayurveda, Unani or Siddha. The anti-colonial history of Naturopathy has been maintained, at least in part, by some members who consider the phenomenon to be a medico-political movement against modernization that advocates for individual freedom and patient empowerment. To them, Naturopathy is a holistic lifestyle that includes a specific political ideology, highly connected to an ecological, democratic and egalitarian way of thinking, as well as an anti-globalization attitude. The continuities of the movement become clear in the explicit target of its political activities: Biopower in the form of pharmaceutical medications, manufactured and endorsed by multi-national Western companies and governments.

© KONINKLIJKE BRILL NV, LEIDEN, 2016 | DOI 10.1163/9789004325104_011

The line of conflict concerning structural pluralism (Sujatha 2007) emerges as a particularity of South Indian Naturopathy: A separation of the movement between college-trained Naturopaths (professionals) and non-degree-holders (psycho-nutritionals). At its core, the separation is a question of trying to reform the medical system from within versus trying to overcome the state-determined system altogether. The former are trying to out-compete other state-approved medical systems through the presentation of their practice as empirical, observation-oriented, evidence-based, quantified, low-priced, gentle, and low-commercialized but still indigenous and local enough to awaken patriotic sentiments in their patients. Their ambition is to institutionalize their particular interpretation of Naturopathy in order to acquire legitimacy and funding by AYUSH, the governmental body responsible for officially legitimizing medical systems and distributing resources to them.

At the same time, there are many practitioners who refuse to have their treatments standardized and institutionalized. One contingent of this group calls themselves psycho-nutritionals and is active mainly in northern Kerala. Psycho-nutritionals see themselves as operating outside the state-sanctioned system of medicine. They understand their interpretation of Naturopathy to fall in the tradition of resistance, seeking to provide individual patients access to knowledge and expertise. Both groups present themselves as opposing in their interpretations, goals and methodologies. The analysis of the daily routines in the hospitals confirms their distinct approaches. While professional Naturopaths put the focus on applied substance-related treatments, psycho-nutritional Naturopaths ensure that all patients receive the same treatment that is based upon integration with each other socially as well as with the medico-political aims of the movement. While both focus on nutrition, for the former this references a material form of medicine (prescribed food) while for the latter it constitutes an integral part of a naturopathically-correct lifestyle.

Common Ground

In taking a closer look at the practices, practitioners and especially the patients in both streams of Naturopathy, a common ground becomes evident. The actual hospital practices enacted by professionals and psycho-nutritionals differ only on accentuation. Psycho-nutritionals rely on simplicity and transparency in order to give the patients the opportunity to implement their treatments at home. However, despite the fact that psycho-nutritionals critique the clinical practices of both allopathic hospitals and professional naturopathic adaptations, they still do not offer a distinct alternative to their patients – indeed, the daily routine in both kinds of hospitals is based on doctor's rounds and specific timeframes for treatment sessions.

All the hospitals examined are organized hierarchically, with specialists as decision-makers, hospital and treatment assistants in the mid-level, and cleaning staff at the very bottom of the hierarchy. This reflects a contradiction in the ideologies of psycho-nutritionals: Their claim of an egalitarian, humanistic, and democratic way of healing does not pervade through the stratification in the hospital. Treatment assistants are in most cases not even aware of the fact that psycho-nutritionals follow a political agenda.

Some medical practices such as diagnosis are externalized to an allopathic system of language by both streams of Naturopathy. Naturopathic practitioners consider the treatment of patients to be their central medical activity, rather than the process of diagnosis. Thus, allopathic knowledge becomes common ground for all hospital actors in the delineation of disease origins. Additionally, most naturopathic practitioners, whether from the professional or psycho-nutritional side, do not see a naturopathic way of life as a guiding principle used to manage their own lives. Instead, they personally use nutritional therapy only in the event that they are affected by a disease themselves.

Patients mostly turn to Naturopathy for treatment of chronic ailments that could not be cured by any other medical system they approached. Similar to treatment assistants, patients generally are not aware of the political implications of the psycho-nutritional movement. They do not, as a whole, see any nuances or distinctions within Naturopathy as a medical system itself and therefore regard the naturopathic hospitals equally. Instead, they seek treatment at these institutions for two different reasons: The first group, the financially "better off" patients, believes in a change of lifestyle to heal their mostly minor diseases. They assume that Naturopathy is a gentle method of treatment, and hope that it can be easily incorporated into their everyday lives. Only a small number in this group consult Naturopaths because they are looking for an alternative to allopathic treatment for their life-changing disease. However, patients with "no other option" seek naturopathic treatment because it is financially the only feasible way to receive medical care or to avoid medication or surgery. Patients in both of these groups are disappointed when they leave the hospital and find themselves unable to implement home treatment on a long-term basis, mostly because sharing food is an essential part of sociality in South India. This prompts many naturopathic patients to return to the hospital again. In both streams of Naturopathy, patients' role is to return to the hospital where they become patients again. Their everyday lives outside the hospital keep them from turning into actants. Sick people do not assume agency as promised by the ideology of psycho-nutritionals.

The Anti-Clinic and the Naturopathic Space

In the second part of this book, I stated that Naturopathy as a medical paradigm has been associated in past work with an inversion of the Foucauldian clinic, the so-called anti-clinic (Alter 2004). Yet, the analysis of the empirical material in this book suggests that this is not the case. The presentation of professional Naturopaths conveys ideas of healing that are congruent with the medical norm – relying on allopathic premises. They aim to constantly produce specialist knowledge and delineate themselves from lay practitioners. They have adapted the institutionalized and educational structures of Allopathy. Patients in their hospitals are categorized according to their diseases and symptoms – an organizational style that becomes most obvious in the case of the GNH with their specialty in renal failure. Their conception of the body and the location of diseases implies the development of a clinical gaze, since it is completely absorbed by allopathic structure. Looking at the actual practices of professional Naturopaths, there are no indicators that it is accurate to categorize their profession as an anti-clinic.

Psycho-nutritionals present themselves in a different way. For them the stated goal of treatment is to transfer agency to the patient: The patient should no longer be docile and passive. The psycho-nutritional cure is a movement of people striving to internalize agency with the overall goal of freeing oneself from external forces and dependencies. According to their ideology, a change of diet, a focus on self-restraint and the maintenance of celibacy cause a moral change and therefore increase the agency of the people. Additionally, psycho-nutritionals move away from the idea of a clinical gaze; instead they strive to see the patient as a whole identity, not only as a body consisting of small entities, such as organs affected by diseases. Therefore, they attempt to form a different kind of norm, where power does not emanate from a center such as the government but rather from the people themselves. Empowerment as a superior goal applies basically to the body of the patient and its power to heal itself, without outside intrusion. Thus, Naturopathy conceived of in this manner is an inversive element in the frame of allopathic biopolitics. Normality is therefore grasped in the different sense of the concept of "living a natural life," in which the body is active, and the person as a whole is self-responsible.

Yet, on a theoretical level the conceptualization of Naturopathy as an anti-clinic is deceptive. The psycho-nutritional credo "come a patient, return a doctor" denotes the internalization of technologies of discipline. For Naturopathy to have a continuous, long-term effect, patients need to acquire specialist knowledge on nutrition and applied substance-related treatments. This specialist knowledge is based upon an ultimate lifestyle change consisting of exhaustive self-control, celibacy and asceticism. In comparison to Allopathy with all its complicated terminology, complex technologies and nontransparent specialist fields, naturopathic specialist knowledge is far less complex. However, it nevertheless requires the patient to intensively grapple with it, and it is only after this intense work that patients can potentially integrate naturopathic fundamentals into their everyday life. In this way, Naturopathy places the responsibility for change onto the individual. This characteristic has been critiqued in relation to Allopathy: Specifically, an underlying focus on self-responsibility can serve as a tactic that ultimately allows those in power to ignore the structural reasons that ill health emerges in the first place, and particularly how unequal burdens of disease are borne by certain groups in society. Ironically, despite its anti-colonial rhetoric, in practice Naturopathy operates in a similar manner – placing the responsibility for social change on the individual, thereby conceptualizing the individual as its source. While those in the Naturopathy movement may consider this to be sufficient to actually create change, they risk placing undue burden on already-sick individuals.

Taking the empirical material of this book into account, the inconsistencies between practitioners' behavior inside and outside the hospital attract attention. It seems that for most of them, Naturopathy is seen as a profession more than a lifestyle. The social stratification in hospitals points to a rather unequal distribution of power among the different actors. The ideology does not seem to pervade to the "average" patient who visits a naturopathic hospital in order to cure his or her chronic ailment. This is due to the fact that psycho-nutritionals adapt their hospitals around allopathic premises, e.g. in their way of structuring their daily routine. Patients leaving these hospitals are not empowered in the sense that psycho-nutritionals want them to be. This means that the actual socio-medical practices in the hospitals fail to uphold this oppositional position to the clinic. Due to the strong public pressure and the fierce competition from standardized medical systems, psycho-nutritionals are struggling to promote their simplicity and banish allopathic testing and interruptions.

The interpretation of the ethnographic material presented in this book proposes that naturopathic hospitals constitute a naturopathic space. The conception of the hospital as a space places the focus on the actual diagnostic and treatment practices and how they are differentially applied there as compared to other social settings. Only specific groups have access to the delimited space of the hospital, in which medical practices are defined, implemented and reproduced. Both streams of naturopathic practitioners create spaces in their hospitals that follow significantly different rules than social life in South India normally allows.

While the theoretical conception of the anti-clinic of Naturopathy as a whole fails, empowerment does takes place in other areas of naturopathic treatment that are not necessarily intended by practitioners. First, although a cure may not be in sight for them, patients from the "no other option" group such as Manoj or Shankar can improve or eliminate some of their symptoms in a naturopathic hospital. This at least buys them time to find other solutions. Furthermore, even if they are not able to fully understand the treatment, some of the basics are nevertheless realizable such as the abandonment of substances that are hard for their organs to process. Naturopaths also convincingly promote the importance of integrating exercise into daily life. The last area of empowerment relates to the externalization of the diagnostic process to allopathic practitioners and labs. This provides patients with more agency within the medical context of the hospital than in other systems such as Allopathy or Ayurveda. The attainment of control over the social interpretation of their disease is of particular importance for patients not only in giving them authorship of their own medical biographies, but also for social purposes seemingly unrelated to the medical context (e.g. in the marriage market).

Future Research

The findings in this ethnography pave the way for several potential research directions. First, the specific concept of nature employed by both streams of Naturopathy as an amalgam of post-Enlightenment, Rousseauian flow from Europe to India, accompanied by local markers such as the idealization of coconuts and bananas, has not so far been examined in detail and calls for further investigation. Alter (2004) states that the reason why Naturopathy has been able to flourish to such an extent is its fertile ground in India: the Indian concept of *prakrti* (translated by him to mean the "laws of nature" [ibid: 128]) feature similar ideas of nature and self:

> What may well have made Nature Cure so popular in India around the turn of the last century was its direct, unmediated appeal to 'nature,' understood as a modern concept denoting the purity of many things – the past, precultural and primordial purity, integrated holism – and the way in which this appeal synchronized with the concept of *prakrti* manifest, most clearly, in *Samkhya* philosophy (ibid: 129).

Indeed, this could be a reasonable explanation for the increasing popularity of Naturopathy in India. However, this leaves open the question of whether a similar conception of nature exists in related medical systems such as Ayurveda, Unani and Yoga, the latter being nowadays almost inseparably bound to

Naturopathy. Other explanations for the strong presence of Naturopathy have included, similar to Europe, the periodic emergence of an ecological movement that critiques the over-engineered, "artificial," money- and career-oriented lifestyle. This may be in response to the general social change taking place in Kerala and the subsequent pressure to achieve a lifestyle similar to that of Gulf repatriates or other wealthier groups. However, a high potential for frustration exists given the unfavorable job market in Kerala. There is also a reasonable hypothesis that the increasing role of Naturopathy may be a product of the political climate: Kerala's communist government fosters a culture of critical thinkers who strike and protest against social inequality. I would suggest these questions as pointers for further studies on Naturopathy.

Certainly the structural pluralism (Sujatha 2007) of Naturopathy in South India is not as dichotomous as illustrated in this book. It can only provide information about one stream of non-professionalized Naturopaths. In reference to Gandhi's approach to health, future research on other non-college-trained medical practitioners in India will illuminate how naturopathic practices can be legitimated in different ways. In the same vein, conducting an in-depth study of health-seeking behavior in other local contexts with naturopathic patients and practitioners will contribute to a better understanding of Naturopathy as a worldwide phenomenon. Dr. Vadakkanchery, for example, is running another hospital in Thailand. Additionally, professionals and psychonutritionals conduct naturopathic health camps in the Middle East for Malayalis as well as locals, promoting a naturopathic way of life according to the *panchabutha* elementary concepts. In our contemporary technological times, medical practices and systems are interconnected at a global level and do not operate in isolation. Investigating the diversity of practices within Naturopathy could shed valuable light on how medical systems more broadly are adopted and localized in particular cultural contexts.

Appendix

1   Infrastructure of AYUSH Systems of Medicine

AYUSH Institutions in India in 2010 (AYUSH 2016a)

TABLE 5   *AYUSH Institutions in India in 2010*

Facility	Ayurveda	Unani	Siddha	Yoga	Naturopathy	Homeo-pathy	Sowa-Rigpa	Total
Hospitals	2,458	269	275	4	24	245	2	3,277
Beds	44,820	4,894	2,576	35	661	9631	32	62,649
Registered practitioners	478,750	51,067	7,195	0	1,401	246,772	0	785,185
UG Colleges	254	39	7	0	10	158	0	495
PG Colleges	64	6	3	0	0	33	0	106

AYUSH Institutions in Kerala in 2010 (AYUSH 2016b)

TABLE 6   *AYUSH Institutions in Kerala in 2010*

Facility	Ayurveda	Unani	Siddha	Yoga	Naturopathy	Homeo-pathy	Sowa-Rigpa	Total
Hospitals	126	0	2	0	2	32	0	162
Beds	4,037	0	170	0	40	1,105	0	5,352
Registered practitioners	16,639	70	1,401	0	0	10,235	0	28,345
UG Colleges	16	0	1	0	0	5	0	22
PG Colleges	82	0	0	0	0	36	0	118

© KONINKLIJKE BRILL NV, LEIDEN, 2016 | DOI 10.1163/9789004325104_012

2   Infrastructure of Naturopathy in India

Naturopathic Hospitals, Total Hospital Beds and Clinics (AYUSH 2016c)

TABLE 7   *Naturopathic Hospitals, Total Hospital Beds and Clinics*

Inpatient Hospitals	About 250 with about 10000 beds total
Outpatient Clinics	About 300 throughout India
Yoga Hospitals	6
Manufacturing Units for Naturopathy Equipment	About 40

3   Admission Form in the MNCC

MAHATHMA NATURE CURE CENTRE
TALIPARAMBA   670 141
ADMISSION FORM

ADMN No.	DOA :	TIME :
ROOM No.	DOD :	TIME :

Name of the Patient   --

Sex   (Please ✓)   [M]   [F]   Age:...............

Address   --

Phone No.   --

Father's/Husband's Name   --

Marital Status& No. of Children   --

Occupation

Present Syptoms

History of illness

Family History

Treatments Taken

		Appetite	Rest	Tobacco
		Thirst	Sleep	Alcohol
		Urine	Recreation/Hobby	Tea
		Stools	Sex	Coffee
		Sweat	Veg/Nonveg	Clothing
		Excerceise /Work	Menstruation	Bath

| Date: | Weight | Height CM | Average Weight Kg |
| | | B.P mmHg | Pulse Rate |

DIAGNOSIS

PLEDGE

I hereby declare that the above mentioned datas are true to the best of my knowledge & belief. I wish to be admited here and take treatments for .... days. I shall agree to abide all the rules of the hospital and also pay the bills accordingly . I am responsible for all the changes in my body as the result of this treatment.

Name & Signature of the Patient

Bi-standers Name & Signature

TREATMENTS

Date	Observation	Forenoon (9-30 a.m.)	Afternoon (3 p.m.)	Evening (7 p.m.)

DIET CHART

Date	9 a.m.	Lunch	11 a.m.	1 p.m.	5 p.m.	7 p.m.

FIGURE 12   *Admission Form in the MNCC*

4   Admission Form in the NLH

LiFE HOSPITAL

നേച്ചർ ലൈഫ് ഹോസ്പിറ്റൽ

പാസ്പോർട്ട് ഓഫീസിന് സമീപം, എരഞ്ഞിപ്പാലം, ക്യാപ്റ്റൻ വിക്രം റോഡ്, കോഴിക്കോട്.

ഫോൺ: 0495 – 2761314, 6451314

Op. No. : ....   തീയതി ....

IP. No. : ....

01) പേര് .... വയസ് .... സ്ത്രീ / പുരുഷൻ

02) മേൽവിലാസം ....

..................................., ഫോൺ : (വീട്) .... (ഓഫീസ്) ....

03) ബന്ധപ്പെടേണ്ട വിലാസം :- പേര് ....

വിലാസം .... ഫോൺ ....

04) തൊഴിൽ .... തൊഴിൽ സ്ഥലം ....

05) നേച്ചർ ലൈഫ് ഹോസ്പിറ്റലിൽ വരുവാൻ ഇടയായതെങ്ങിനെ? ....

06) ഏതെങ്കിലും തരത്തിലുള്ള ഓപ്പറേഷൻ വിധേയമായിട്ടുണ്ടോ? ....

07) എക്സറേ, ബയോപ്സി, സ്കാനിങ്ങ്, ഡയാലിസിസ്, രക്തം സ്വീകരിക്കൽ, റേഡിയേഷൻ തുടങ്ങിയവ നടത്തിയിട്ടുണ്ടോ ? എന്തിന് എത്രപ്രാവശ്യം ....

08) ശരീരത്തിൽ ഏതെങ്കിലും വിധ വസ്തുക്കളോ, അവയവങ്ങളോ വെച്ചുപിടിപ്പിച്ചിട്ടുണ്ടോ? ....

09) മത്സ്യം, മാംസം, മുട്ട കഴിക്കുമോ? ....

10) പുകവലി, മദ്യം, മുറുക്ക്, ചായ, കാപ്പി ഇവ ദിവസത്തിൽ എത്രവീതം? എത്രകാലമായി? ....

....

11) ഗർഭാശയ ചികിത്സകൾ ചെയ്തിട്ടുണ്ടോ? എന്തെല്ലാം? ....

12) ഇപ്പോഴുള്ള അസുഖങ്ങൾ എന്തെല്ലാം? ....

13) പാരസെറ്റമോൾ ഗുളികകൾ കഴിക്കാറുണ്ടോ? എപ്പോഴെല്ലാം ? ....

14) ഇപ്പോൾ കഴിച്ചുകൊണ്ടിരിക്കുന്ന മരുന്നുകൾ എന്തെല്ലാം? എത്രകാലമായി ? ....

NATURE LIFE HOSPITAL

Captain Vikram Road, Eranhipalam, Kozhikode - 6

TREATMENT CHART

Name of Patient ....

Date	Enema	ENT Wash	Wet Pack	Sun Bath	Spinal Bath	Hip Bath	Mud Pack	Mud Paste	Kidney Pack	"T" Pack	Eye Pack	Eye Drops	Eye Exercise	Herbal Paste	Hip Bath (Hot Water)	Spinal Bath (Hot)	Special Enema	Massage	Steam Bath	Inhalation	Yoga	Hot & Cold	Head Wash	Others

NATURE LIFE HOSPITAL & REMEDIES
DIET CHART

Date	6 00 AM	8 30 AM	10 30 AM	12 30 PM	3 30 PM	6 00 PM	NP1

FIGURE 13   *Admission Form in the NLH*

Translation of the admission form in the NLH (Indu P.):

Date:

1) Name: Age: Gender:
2) Address:
   Phone:
3) Permanent Address:
4) Profession:
5) What is the reason for coming to the Nature Life Hospital?
6) Have you had any surgeries?
7) Have you had an X-ray, scanning, biopsy, dialysis, radiation, etc. performed?
8) Do you have any transplanted organs?
9) Do you eat meat, fish or eggs?
10) Do you smoke, drink alcohol, tea or coffee? How often?
11) Did you receive any treatment for pregnancy?
12) What are your current diseases?
13) Are you taking Paracetamol tablets?
14) Which medicines are you taking at present? How often?
15) Describe all the diseases and treatments that you have had since birth.

(the following text is dictated by the responsible doctor registering the patient in the NLH:*)*

I understand the treatment of Naturopathy. I am ready to stay here and I am allowing my body to be treated. If I am not following the diet and if any harm happens to my body during the time of the treatment I am responsible for that. Signature:

Bibliography

Aanaiappan, M. *How to Cure Diseases with Natural Foods?* 2 vols. Hyderabad: Good Health Foundation, 1999-2000.

Addlakha, Renu. *Deconstructing Mental Illness: An Ethnography of Psychiatry, Women and the Family.* New Delhi: Zubaan Books, 2008.

Agic, Haris. "Hope Rites: An Ethnographic Study of Mechanical Help-Heart Implantation Treatment." Ph.D. diss., Linköping University, 2012.

Alex, Gabriele. *Medizinische Diversität im Postkolonialen Indien: Dynamik und Perzeption von Gesundheitsangeboten in Tamil Nadu.* Berlin: Weißenseeverlag, 2010.

Allard, James Robert. *Romanticism, Medicine, and the Poet's Body.* London: Ashgate, 2007.

Alter, Joseph S, ed. *Asian Medicine and Globalization.* Philadelphia: University of Pennsylvania Press, 2005.

Alter, Joseph S, ed. *Gandhi's Body: Sex, Diet, and the Politics of Nationalism.* Philadelphia: University of Pennsylvania Press, 2000.

Alter, Joseph S, ed. "Nature Cure and Ayurveda: Nationalism, Viscerality and Bio-ecology in India." In: *Body & Society* 21, no. 1 (2015): 3-28.

Alter, Joseph S, ed. *Yoga in Modern India: The Body between Science and Philosophy.* Princeton: Princeton University Press, 2004.

Alter, Joseph S, ed. "Yoga, Modernity and the Middle-Class: Locating the Body in a World of Desire." In *A Companion to South Asian Studies*, edited by Isabelle Clark-Deces. Oxford: Wiley-Blackwell, 2011.

Andersen, Helle Max. "'Villagers' Differential Treatment in a Ghanaian Hospital." In *Social Science and Medicine* 59 (2004): 2003-12.

Appadurai, Arjun. "Disjuncture and Difference in the Global Cultural Economy." In *The Anthropology of Globalization: A Reader*, edited by Jonathan Xavier Inda and Renato Rosaldo. Malden: Wiley-Blackwell, 2002.

Appadurai, Arjun. "How to Make a National Cuisine: Cookbooks in Contemporary India." In *Food and Culture: A Reader*, edited by Carole Counihan and Penny van Esterik. New York: Routledge, 1997.

Appadurai, Arjun. *Modernity at Large: Cultural Dimensions of Globalization.* Minneapolis: University of Minnesota Press, 1996.

Arnold, David. *Colonizing the Body: State Medicine and Epidemic Disease in Nineteenth-Century India.* Berkeley: University of California Press, 1993.

Arnold, David, ed. *Imperial Medicine and Indigenous Societies.* New Delhi: Oxford University Press, 1989.

Arnold, David. *The New Cambridge History of India: Science, Technology and Medicine in Colonial India.* Cambridge: Cambridge University Press, 2000.

AYUSH. "1.1 Summary of Infrastructure Facilities under AYUSH." Accessed February 2016a. Ministry of AYUSH, AYUSH Bhawan, B Block, GPO Complex, INA, New Delhi <http://www.indianmedicine.nic.in/showfile.asp?lid=44>.

AYUSH. "Kerala." Accessed Februaury 2016b. Ministry of AYUSH, AYUSH Bhawan, B Block, GPO Complex, INA, New Delhi <http://www.indianmedicine.nic.in/writereaddata/linkimages/3979851858-Kerala.pdf>.

AYUSH. "Naturopathy Specialty Centers." Accessed February 2016c. Ministry of AYUSH, AYUSH Bhawan, B Block, GPO Complex, INA, New Delhi <http://www.indianmedicine.nic.in/index3.asp?sslid=276&subsublinkid=93&lang=1>.

AYUSH. "Welcome to AYUSH." Accessed February 2016d. Ministry of AYUSH, AYUSH Bhawan, B Block, GPO Complex, INA, New Delhi <http://indianmedicine.nic.in/index.asp?lang=1>.

AINCF. "Dr. Brij Bhushan Goel: All India Nature Cure Ferderation (A Non-Profit Organisation). Accessed February 2016 <http://lifehappy.org/content/profile/aincf.asp>.

Baby, John. *Correct Nutrients Cure Diseases*. N.p., 2004.

Baby, John. *Principles and Procedures of Drugless Cure*. N.p., 2010.

Baer, Hans. *The Sociopolitical Status of U.S. Naturopathy at the Dawn of the Twenty-First Century*. In *Medical Anthropology Quarterly*, 15, no. 3 (2001): 329-346.

Baer, Hans and Stephen Sporn. *Naturopathy Around the World: Variations and Political Dilemmas of an Eclectic Heterodox Medical System*. New York: Nova Science Publishers, 2009.

Banerjee, Abhradip, Gopalkrishna Chakrabarti and Arnab Das. "A New Beginning in Medical Anthropology: Scope and Relevance of 'Pharmaceutical Anthropology' in India." In *Euras J Anthropol* 4, no. 2 (2013):51-57.

Banerji, Chitrita. *Eating India: Exploring the Food and Culture of the Land of Spices*. London: Bloomsbury Publishing, 2010.

Banerjee, Madhulika. "Local Knowledge for World Market: Globalising Ayurveda." In *Economic and Political Weekly* 39, no. 1 (2004): 89-93.

Beal, Allan R. "Strategies of Resort to Curers in South India." In *Asian Medical Systems*, edited by Charles M. Leslie. Berkeley: University of California Press, 1976.

Beckenridge, Carol, ed. *Consuming Modernity: Public Culture in a South Asian World*. Minneapolis: University of Minnesota Press, 1995.

Bode, Marteen. "Taking Traditional Knowledge to the Market: The Commoditization of Indian Medicine." In *Anthropology and Medicine* 13, no. 3 (2006): 225-236.

Bode, Marteen. *Taking Traditional Knowledge to the Market: The Modern Image of the Ayurvedic and Unani Industry 1980-2000*. Hyderabad: Orient Blackswan Pvt Ltd, 2008.

Brass, Paul. "The Politics of Ayurvedic Education: A Case Study of Revivalism and Modernization in India." In *Education and Politics in India: Studies in Organization,*

Society and Policy, edited by Susanne Hoeber Rudolph and Lloyd I. Rudolph. Cambridge: Harvard University Press, 1972.

Brimnes, Niels. "The Sympathizing Heart and the Healing Hand: Smallpox Prevention and Medical Benevolence in Early Colonial South India." In *Colonialism as Civilizing Mission: Cultural Ideology in British India*, edited by Harald Fischer-Tiné and Michael Mann. London: Anthem Press, 2004.

Brosius, Christiane. *India's Middle Class: New Forms of Urban Leisure, Consumption and Prosperity*. New Delhi: Routledge, 2010.

Brown, H. "Hospital Domestics Care Work in a Kenyan Hospital." In *Space and Culture* 15, no. 1 (2012): 18-30.

Brown, Judith. *Gandhi: Prisoner of Hope*. New Haven: Yale University Press, 1989.

Cassidy, Claire. "Social Science Theory and Methods in the Study of Alternative and Complementary Medicine." In *The Journal of Alternative and Complementary Medicine* 1, no. 1 (1995): 19–40.

Caudill, William. *The Psychiatric Hospital as a Small Community*. Cambridge: Harvard University Press, 1958.

CCIM (Central Council of Indian Medicine). Accessed February 2016 <http://www.ccimindia.org/>.

CCRYN (Central Council for Research in Yoga & Naturopathy). Accessed February 2016 <http://www.ccryn.org/>.

Chacko, Elisabeth. "Culture and Therapy: Complementary Strategies for the Treatment of Type-2 Diabetes in an Urban Setting in Kerala, India." In *Social Science and Medicine* 56, no. 5 (2003): 1087-98.

Charis Holistic Center. "Psycho-Nutrition: Starving the Mind or Feeding it?", blog entry by Barbara Charis, February 9, 2012. Accessed February 2016 <http://blog.charisholisticcenter.com/2012/02/09/psycho-nutrition-starving-the-mind-or-feeding-it.aspx>.

Chenhall, Richard. "What's in a Rehab? Ethnographic Evaluation Research in Indigenous Australian Residential Alcohol and Drug Rehabilitation Centres." In *Anthropology and Medicine* 15, no. 2 (2008): 105-116.

Cherukara, Joseph M. and James Manalel. "Medical Tourism in Kerala: Challenges and Scope." Paper presented at the Conference on Tourism in India: Challenges Ahead, Kozhikode, 15-17 May 2008.

Chua, Jocelyn Lim. *In Pursuit of the Good Life: Aspiration and Suicide in Globalizing South India*. Berkeley: University of California Press, 2014.

Connor, Linda and Geoffrey Samuel, eds. *Healing Powers and Modernity: Traditional Medicine, Shamanism and Science in Asian Societies*. Westport: Bergin and Garvey, 2001.

Coser, Rose L. *Life in the Ward*. East Lansing: Michigan State University Press, 1962.

Cyranski, Christoph. "Oil Massages, Purges and Beach Holidays: Ayurvedic Health Tourism in Kerala, South India." PhD diss., Heidelberg University, forthcoming.

Das, Ratan. *The Global Vision of Mahatma Gandhi*. New Delhi: Sarup & Sons, 2005.

Delhi Medical Council. Accessed February 2016 <http://delhimedicalcouncil.nic.in/>.

Dhanda, Amita. *Legal Order and Mental Disorder*. New Delhi: Sage Publications, 2000.

Dreyfus, Hubert and Paul Rabinow. *Michel Foucault: Jenseits von Strukturalismus und Hermeneutik*. Frankfurt am Main: Athenäum Verlag, 1987.

Dunn, Frederick. "Traditional Asian Medicine and Cosmopolitan Medicine as Adaptive Systems." In *Asian Medical Systems*, edited by Charles Leslie, Berkeley: University of California Press, 1976.

Ecks, Stefan. "Bodily Sovereignty as Political Sovereignty: 'Self-care' in Kolkata (India)." In *Anthropology and Medicine* 11, no. 1 (2004): 75-89.

Ecks, Stefan. *Eating Drugs: Psychopharmaceutical Pluralism in India*. New York: New York University Press, 2013.

Ecks, Stefan. *Mind Food: Plural Mood Medications in India*. New York: New York University Press, forthcoming.

Ecks, Stefan. "Pharmaceutical Citizenship: Antidepressant Marketing and the Promise of Demarginalization in India." In *Anthropology and Medicine* 12, no. 3 (2005): 239-254.

Engler, Steven. "'Science' vs. 'Religion' in Classical Ayurveda." In *Numen* 50, no. 4 (2003): 416-463.

Erikson, Erik. *Gandhi's Truth. On the Origins of Militant Nonviolence*. New York: Norton & Company, 1969.

Farquhar, Judith. *Knowing Practice: The Clinical Encounter of Chinese Medicine*. Boulder: Westview Press, 1994.

Fernandes, Leela. *India's New Middle Class: Democratic Politics in an Era of Economic Reform*. Minneapolis: University of Minnesota Press, 2006.

Finkler, Katja. "Biomedicine Globalized and Localized: Western Medical Practices in an Outpatient Clinic of a Mexican Hospital." In *Social Science and Medicine* 59, no. 10 (2004): 2037-51.

First Post India. "HDI in India rises by 21%: Kerala leads, Gujarat far behind." Published October 21, 2011. Accessed February 2016 <http://www.firstpost.com/india/hdi-in-india-rises-by-21-kerala-leads-gujarat-far-behind-114044.html>.

Foucault, Michel. *The Birth of the Clinic: An Archaeology of Medical Perception*. New York: Pantheon Books, 1973.

Foucault, Michel. *Discipline and Punish: The Birth of the Prison*. New York: Vintage, 1977.

Foucault, Michel. "Of Other Spaces." Translated by Jay Miskowiec. In *Diacritics* 16, no. 1 (1986): 22-27.

Foucault, Michel. *Power/Knowledge: Selected Interviews and Other Writings, 1972-1977*. Edited by Colin Gordon. New York: Pantheon Books, 1980.

Frank, Robert. *Globalisierung 'Alternativer' Medizin: Homöopathie und Ayurveda in Deutschland und Indien*. Bielefeld: Transcript, 2004.

Fuller, Christopher and Haripriya Narasimhan. "Information Technology Professionals and the New-Rich Middle Class in Chennai (Madras)." In *Modern Asian Studies* 41, no. 1 (2007): 121-50.

Gaines, Atwood and Robert Hahn, eds. *Physicians of Western Medicine: Anthropological Approaches to Theory and Practice.* Dordrecht: D. Reidel Publishing, 1985.

Gandhi, Mahatma. *An Autobiography or The Story of my Experiments with Truth.* Ahmedabad: Navajivan Publishing House, 2013. First published 1927.

Gandhi, Mahatma. *Diet and Diet Reform.* Ahmedabad: Navajivan Publishing House, 1949.

Gandhi, Mahatma. *A Guide to Health.* Translated by A. Rama Iyer. Madras: S. Ganesan Publisher, 1921.

Gandhi, Mahatma. *Indian Home Rule.* Phoenix: The International Printing Press, 1909.

Gandhi, Mahatma. *Key to Health.* Ahmedabad: Navajivan Publishing House, 1948.

Ganguly-Scrase, Ruchira and Timothy Scrase. *Globalisation and the Middle Classes in India: The Social and Cultural Impact of Neoliberal Reforms.* London: Routledge, 2009.

Geertsen, Reed, Melville R. Klauber, Mark Rindflesh, Robert L. Kane and Robert Grey. "A Re-examination of Suchman's View on Social Factors in Health Care Utilization." *Journal of Health and Social Behavior* 16, no. 2 (1975): 226-37.

Geest, Sijaak van der and Katja Finkler: "Hospital Ethnography: Introduction." In *Social Science and Medicine* 59, no. 10 (2004): 1995- 2001.

Geest, Sijaak van der and Samuel Sarkodie. "The Fake Patients: A Research Experiment in a Ghanian Hospital." In *Social Science and Medicine* 47, no. 9 (1999): 1373-81.

Geest, Sijaak van der, Susan Reynolds Whyte and Anita Hardon. "The Anthropology of Pharmaceuticals: A Biographical Approach." In *Annual Review of Anthropology* 25, (October 1996): 153-78.

Gibson, D. "The Gaps in the Gaze in South African Hospitals." In *Social Science and Medicine* 59, no. 10 (2004): 2013-24.

Goffman, Erving. *Asylums: Essays on the Social Situation of Mental Patients and Other Inmates.* New York: Doubleday Anchor, 1961.

Good, Byron J. *Medicine, Rationality and Experience: An Anthropological Perspective.* Cambridge: Cambridge University Press, 1994.

Good, Mary-Jo D. "Cultural Studies of Biomedicine: An Agenda for Research." In *Social Science and Medicine* 41, no. 4 (1995): 461-73.

Good, Byron J. and Mary-Jo D. Good. "The Cultural Context of Diagnosis and Therapy: A View from Medical Anthropology." In *Mental Health Resource and Practice in Minority Communities.* Edited by M. Miranda. Washington: U.S. Department of Health and Human Services, 1986, 1-27.

Gopinath, N. "Nutrition and Chronic Diseases – Indian Experience." In *Southeast Asian Journal of Tropical Medicine and Public Health* 28, no. 2 (1997): 113–17.

Gupta, R. "Burden of Coronary Heart Disease in India." In *Indian Heart Journal* 57, no. 6 (2005): 632-38.

Hackett, Latha and Richard Hackett. "Coconuts and Conduct Disorder: Child Psychiatry in Kerala?" In *Psychiatric Bulletin* 14, no. 7 (1990): 422-424.

Hahn, Robert A. and Arthur Kleinman. "Biomedical Practice and Anthropological Theory: Frameworks and Directions." In *Annual Review of Anthropology* 12, (October 1983): 305-33.

Halliburton, Murphy. "The Importance of a Pleasant Process of Treatment: Lessons on Healing from South India." In *Culture, Medicine and Psychiatry* 27, no. 2 (2003): 161-86.

Halliburton, Murphy. *Mudpacks and Prozac: Experiencing Ayurvedic, Biomedical, and Religious Healing*. Walnut Creek: Left Coast Press, 2009.

Halliburton, Murphy. "Possession, Purgatives or Prozac? The Experience of Illness and the Process of Healing in Kerala, South India." PhD diss., University of New York, 2000.

Halliburton, Murphy. "Suicide: A Paradox of Development in Kerala." In *Economic and Political Weekly* 33, no. 36-37 (1998): 2341-45.

Harrison, Mark. "Medicine and Orientalism: Perspectives in Europe's Encounter with Indian Medical Systems." In *Health, Medicine and the Empire: Perspectives on Colonial India*. Edited by Biswamoy Pati and Mark Harrison. Hyderabad: Orient Longman, 2001.

Hausmann-Muela, Susanna, Joan Muela Ribera and Isaac Nyamongo, Isaac. "Health Seeking Behaviour and the Health System Response." In *Disease Control Working Paper* 14 (August 2003), Bethesda: Disease Control Priority Project.

Heyll, Uwe. *Wasser, Fasten, Luft und Licht: Die Geschichte der Naturheilkunde in Deutschland*. Frankfurt am Main: Campus, 2006.

Hörbst, Viola and Angelika Wolf. "ARVs and ARTs: Medicoscapes and the Unequal Place-making for Biomedical Treatments in sub-Saharan Africa." In *Medical Anthropology Quarterly* 28, no. 2 (2014): 182-202.

Hörbst, Viola and Angelika Wolf, eds. *Medizin und Globalisierung: Universelle Ansprüche – Lokale Antworten*. Münster: LIT, 2003.

Hörbst, Viola and Kristine Krause. ",On the move' – Die Globalisierungsdebatte in der Medizinethnologie." In *Curare* 27, no. 1 and 2 (2004): 41-60.

Horden, Peregrine. Introduction to *The Body in Balance: Humoral Medicines in Practice*, edited by Peregrine Horden and Elisabeth Hsu. Oxford: Berghahn Books, 2013.

INYGMA. Accessed February 2016 <http://inygmakerala.blogspot.com/>.

Jain, Sumeet and Susrut Jadhav. "Pills that Swallow Policy: Clinical Ethnography of a Community Mental Health Program in Northern India." In *Transcultural Psychiatry* 46, no. 1 (2009): 60–85.

Jannabhumi Daily. "Teacher Made a Student a Guinea Pig by Conducting Naturopathy Treatment for Cancer." May 22, 2005. Translated by Indu P.

Jaye, Chrystal, Tony Egan and Sarah Parker. "'Do as I Say, Not as I Do': Medical Education and Foucault's Normalizing Technologies of Self." In *Anthropology and Medicine* 13, no. 2 (2006): 141-155.

Jeffrey, Robin. *Politics, Women and the Well-being: How Kerala Became a "Model".* New Delhi: Oxford University Press, 1993.

Jenkins, Tania M. "Who is the Boss? Diagnosis and Medical Authority." In *Social Issues in Diagnosis: An Introduction for Students and Clinicans*, edited by A. Jutel and K. Dew. Baltimore: Johns Hopkins University Press, 2014.

Jindal Naturecure Institute. Accessed February 2016 <http://jindalnaturecure.org/>.

Jindal, Rakesh. *Science of Natural Life: A Complete and Easy Book on Nature Cure Principles, Methods and Experiments on Almost All Diseases with Photographs.* New Delhi: Balaji Offset, 2002.

Jungborn Harz. Accessed February 2016 <http://www.jungborn-harz.eu/index. php?menuid=1/>.

Jussuwalla, J. M. *Healing from Within: A Treatise on the Philosophy and Therapy of Nature Cure.* Bombay: Manaktalas, 1956.

Just, Adolf. *Return to Nature: Paradise Regained.* Pomeroy: Health Research, 1996. Copyrighted 1903.

Justice, Judith. *Policies, Plans, and People: Foreign Aid and Health Development.* Berkeley: University of California Press, 1989.

Kaiser, Ronald. *Die Professionalisierung der Ayurvedischen Medizin und deren Rolle im Indischen Medizinpluralismus.* Bonn: Holos Verlag, 1992.

Kakar, Sudhir. *Intimate Relations: Exploring Indian Sexuality.* Chicago: University of Chicago Press, 1990.

Kalayam, Ashraf. "Psychonutritional Cure Methods in the Cure Process of Type 2 Diabetes Mellitus." PhD diss., University of Calicut, 2008.

King, Helen. "Female Fluids in the Hippocratic Corpus: How Solid was the Humoral Body?" In *The Body in Balance: Humoral Medicines in Practise*, edited by Peregrine Horden and Elisabeth Hsu. Oxford: Berghahn Books, 2013.

Kirchfeld, Friedhelm and Wade Boyle. *Nature Doctors: Pioneers in Naturopathic Medicine.* Portland: NCNM Press, 1994.

Kirmayer, L. "Cultural Variations in the Response to Psychiatric Disorders and Emotional Distress." In *Social Science and Medicine* 29, no. 3 (1989): 327-39.

Kleinman, Arthur. *Patients and Healers in the Context of Culture: An Exploration of the Borderland between Anthropology, Medicine, and Psychiatry.* Berkeley: University of California Press, 1980.

Kneipp. "The Five Pillars." Accessed February 2016. https://web.archive.org/web/20151117184131/http://kneippus.com/five-pillars.html

Kneipp, Sebastian. *My Water-Cure.* Whitefish: Kessinger Pub, 2003. First published 1886.

Kneippbund. Accessed February 2016 <http://www.kneippbund.de/>.

Kneipp-Journal. "Ein Denkwürdiges Jubiläum. Die Fünf Elemente des Gesundheitssystems nach Kneipp." Juni, 2010.

Kröger, Alex. "Anthropological and Socio-Medical Health Care Research in Developing Countries." In *Social Sciences and Medicine* 17, no. 3 (1983): 147-61.

Kuhne, Louis. *Neo Naturopathy: The New Science of Healing or the Doctrine of Unity of Diseases.* Whitefish: Kessinger Pub, 2003. Fist published 1899.

Kuhne, Louis. *The Science of Facial Expression.* Whitefish: Kessinger Pub, 2010. First published 1917.

Kumar, Deepak. "Medical Encounters in British India 1820 – 1920." In *Economic and Political Weekly* 32, no. 4 (1997): 166-70.

Kumar, Harilakshmeendra. "Nature Cure: The Original Health Care System: A Critique." PhD diss., Kottayam Mahatma Gandhi University, 2005.

Lambert, Helen: "Evidentiary Truths? The Evidence of Anthropology through the Anthropology of Medical Evidence." In *Anthropology Today* 25, no. 1 (2009): 16-20.

Lang, Claudia. "Trick or Treat? Muslim Thangals, Psychologisation and Pragmatic Realism in Northern Kerala, India." In *Transcultural Psychiatry* 5, no. 6 (2014): 904-923.

Lang, Claudia and Eva Jansen. "The Ayurvedic Appropriation of Depression: Biomedicalizing Ayurvedic Psychiatry in Kerala, India." In *Medical Anthropology*, 32, no. 1 (2013): 25-45.

Lang, Claudia and Eva Jansen. "Depression und die Revitalisierung der Ayurvedischen Psychiatrie in Kerala, Indien." In *Curare* 33, no. 3 and 4 (2010).

Langford, Jean. *Fluent Bodies: Ayurvedic Remedies for Postcolonial Imbalance.* Durham: Duke University Press, 2002.

Langwick, Stacey A. "Articulate(d) Bodies: Traditional Medicine in a Tanzanian Hospital." In *American Ethnologist* 35, no. 3 (2008): 428-439.

Leslie, Charles. *Asian Medical Systems: A Comparative Study.* Berkeley: University of California Press, 1976.

Leslie, Charles. "The Professionalization of Ayurvedic and Unani Medicine." In *Medical Professionals and the Organization of Knowledge,* edited by Eliot Freidson and Judith Lorber. New Brunswick: AldineTransaction, 1972.

Leslie, Charles and Allan Young, eds. *Paths to Asian Medical Knowledge.* Berkeley: University of California Press, 1992.

Liebeskind, Claudia. "Unani Medicine of the Subkontinent." In *Oriental Medicine: An Illustrated Guide to the Asian Arts of Healing,* edited by Jan van Alphen and Anthony Aris. London: Serindia Publications, 1995.

Liechty, Mark. *Suitable Modern: Making Middle-Class Culture in a New Consumer Society.* Princeton: Princeton University Press, 2003.

Lindenbaum, Shirley and Margaret Lock, eds. *Knowledge, Power and Practice: The Anthropology of Medicine and Everyday Life.* Berkeley: University of California Press, 1993.

Livingston, Julie. *Improvising Medicine: An African Oncology Ward in an Emerging Cancer Epidemic*. Durham: Duke University Press, 2012.

Long, Debbi, Cynthia Hunter and Sjaak van der Geest. "Introduction: When the Field is a Ward or a Clinic: Hospital Ethnography." In *Anthropology and Medicine* 15, no. 2 (2008): 71-78.

Löwy, Michael. "The Romantic and the Marxist Critique of Modern Civilization." In *Theory and Society* 16, no. 6 (1987): 891-904.

Malayalam Manorama. "Students Protesting Against the Introduction of B-class Registration." February 4, 2011. Translated by Indu P.

Marcus, George A. "Ethnography in/of the World System: The Emergence of Multi-Sited Ethnography." In *Annual Review of Anthropology* 24 (1995): 95-117.

Martens, Pim. "Health Transitions in a Globalising World: Towards More Disease or Sustained Health?" In *Futures* 34, no. 7 (2002): 635-648.

Math, Suresh Bada, C. R. Chandrashekar and Dinesh Bhugra. "Psychiatric Epidemiology in India." In *Indian Journal of Medical Research* 126, no. 3 (2007): 183-192.

Mathew, E. T. *Employment and Unemployment in Kerala: Some Neglected Aspects*. New Delhi: Sage Publications, 1997.

MDNIY. Accessed February 2016 <http://www.yogamdniy.com/>.

MHCB. "Mental Health Care Bill, 2013." Accessed February 2016 <http://www.prsindia. org/administrator/uploads/general/1376983253~~mental%20health%20care%20 bill%202013.pdf>.

Ministry of Health and Family Welfare. Accessed February 2016 <http://mohfw.nic.in/>.

Mittal, Mahendra. *The Essence of the Vedas*. New Delhi: Manoj Publications, 2005.

Mol, Annemarie. *The Body Multiple: Ontology in Medical Practice*. Durham: Duke University Press, 2002.

Mol, Annemarie. *The Logic of Care: Health and the Problem of Patient Choice*. New York: Routledge, 2008.

Mukharji, Projit B. *Nationalizing the Body: The Market, Print and Daktari Medicine*, London: Anthem Press, 2011.

Nair, Pradeep and Awantika Nanda. "Naturopathic Medicine in India." In *Focus on Alternative and Complementary Therapies* 19, no. 3 (2014): 140-147.

Nanda, B. R. *In Search of Gandhi: Essays and Reflections*. New Delhi: Oxford University Press, 2002.

Naraindas, Harish. "Of Relics, Body Parts and Laser Beams: The German Heilpraktiker and his Ayurvedic Spa." In *Anthropology and Medicine* 18, no. 1 (2011): 67-86.

Naraindas, Harish. "Of Spineless Babies and Folic Acid: Evidence and Efficacy in Biomedicine and Ayurvedic Medicine." In *Social Science and Medicine* 62, no. 11 (2006): 2658-69.

Nichter, Mark. "Paying for What Ails You: Sociocultural Issues Influencing the Ways and Means of Therapy Payment in South India." In *Anthropology and International Health:*

Asian Case Studies, edited by Mark Nichter and Mimi Nichter. Amsterdam: Gordon and Breach, 1996.

Nichter, Mark. "The Political Ecology of Health in India: Indigestion as Sign and Symptom of Defective Modernisation." In *Healing Powers and Modernity: Traditional Medicine, Shamanism and Science in Asian Societies*, edited by Linda H. Connor and Geoffrey Samuel. London: Bergin and Garvey, 2001.

Nichter, Mark. "The Primary Health Center as a Social System: Primary Health Care, Social Status, and the Issue of Team-Work in South Asia." In *Social Science and Medicine* 23, no. 4 (1986): 347-355.

Nichter, Mark. "The Social Relations of Therapy Management." In *New Horizons in Medical Anthropology: Essays in Honour of Charles Leslie*, edited by Mark Nichter and Margret Lock. London: Routledge, 2002.

National Institute of Naturopathy. Accessed February 2016 <http://www.punenin.org/>.

Nisargopachar. "Cry Not on Accidents. Detoxify for Health." Vol. 17, no. 1 (2009a): 24.

Nisargopachar. "Naturopathy and Yoga Therapists's Advice" Vol. 2, no. 2 (2010b): 14.

Nisargopachar. "Naturopathy and Yoga Therapists's Advice" Vol. 2, no. 8 (2010c): 12.

Norwood, Frances. "The Ambivalent Chaplain: Negotiating Structural and Ideological Difference on the Margins of Modern-Day Hospital Medicine." In *Medical Anthropology* 25, no. 1 (2006): 1-29.

Obrist, Birgit. "Medicalization and Morality in a Weak State: Health, Hygiene and Water in Dar Es Salaam, Tanzania." In *Anthropology and Medicine* 11, no. 1 (2004): 43-57.

Oerlemans, Onno. *Romanticism and the Materiality of Nature*. Toronto: University of Toronto Press, 2002.

Osella, Filippo and Caroline Osella. "Food, Memory, Community: Kerala as both 'Indian Ocean' Zone and as Agricultural Homeland." In *South Asia Journal of South Asian Studies* 31, no. 1 (2008): 170-198.

Osella, Filippo and Caroline Osella. "'I am Gulf': The Production of Cosmopolitanism among the Koyas of Kozhikode, Kerala." In *Struggling with History: Islam and Cosmopolitanism in the Western Indian Ocean*, edited by Edward Simpson and Kai Kresse. New York: Columbia University Press, 2007.

Osella, Filippo and Caroline Osella. *Social Mobility in Kerala: Modernity and Identity in Conflict*. London: Pluto Press, 2000.

Palekar, Subhash. *Zero Budget Natural Farming: The Philosophy of Spiritual Farming*. Amravati: Atharva Publications, n.d.

Prakash, Gyan. *Bonded Histories: Genealogies of Labor Servitude in Colonial India*. Cambridge: Cambridge University Press, 1990.

Priya, Ritu. "AYUSH and Public Health: Democratic Pluralism and the Quality of Health Services." In *Medical Pluralism in Contemporary India*, edited by V. Sujatha and Leena Abraham. New Delhi: Orient Blackswan, 2012.

Prost, Audrey. *Precious Pills: Medicine and Social Change among Tibetan Refugees in India*. New York: Berghahn Books, 2008.

Quack, Johannes. "Ignorance and Utilization: Mental Health Care Outside the Purview of the Indian State." In *Anthropology and Medicine* 19, no. 3 (2012): 277-290.

Quack, Johannes and Ananda S. Chopra. "Asymmetrical Translations of Biomedicine in India: The Cases of Contemporary Āyurveda and Psychiatry." In *Vienna Ethnological Newsletter* 13, no. 2-3 (2011): 13-24.

Quaiser, Neshat. "Unani Medical Culture: Memory, Representation, and the Literate Critical Anticolonial Public Sphere." In *Contesting Colonial Authority: Medicine and Indigenous Responses in 19th and 20th-Century India*, edited by Poonam Bala. Lanham: Lexington Books, 2012a.

Quaiser, Neshat. "Tension, Placation, Complaint: Unani and Post-Colonial Medical Communalism." In *Medical Pluralism in Contemporary India*, edited by V. Sujatha and Leena Abraham. Hyderabad: Orient Blackswan, 2012b.

Rabinow, Paul and Nikolas Rose. "Biopower Today." In *BioSocieties* 1,(2006): 195-217.

Radhakrishnan, P. "Land reforms and social change: Study of a Kerala Village." In *Economic and Political Weekly* 18, no. 52-53 (1983): 24-31.

Rajiv Gandhi University. RULES FOR *B.N.Y.S.* Unpublished syllabus, available in the College. Bangalore, 2011 (year of purchase).

Rhodes, L. A. "Studying Biomedicine as a Cultural System." In *Medical Anthropology: A Handbook of Theory and Method*, edited by T. B. Johnson and C. F. Sargent. New York: Greenwood Press, 1990.

Robertson, Roland. *Globalization: Social Theory and Global Culture*. London: Sage Publications, 1992.

Rosenhan, David L. "On Being Sane in Insane Places." In *The Art of Medical Anthropology: Readings*, edited by Sjaak Van der Geest and Adri Rienks. Amsterdam: Het Spinhuis, 1998.

Rothermund, Dietmar. *Mahatma Gandhi*. München: C. H. Beck, 2003.

Salkeld, Ellen J. "Framework Negotiations: Diagnostic Insights among Alternative Medical Practitioners Participating in Integrative Medicine Case Conferences." In *Medical Anthropology Quarterly* 28, no. 1 (2014): 44-65.

Samuelsen, Helle and Vibeke Steffen. "The Relevance of Foucault and Bourdieu for Medical Anthropology: Exploring New Sites." In *Anthropology and Medicine* 11, no. 1 (2004): 3-10.

Sarkar, Tanika. "Gandhi and Social Relations." In *The Cambridge Companion to Gandhi*, edited by Judith M. Brown and Anthony Parel. Cambridge: Cambridge University Press, 2011.

Sarma, Lakshmana K. and S. Swaminathan. *Speaking of Nature Cure: Regain and Improve Health the Drugless Way*. Pudukkottai: The Nature Cure Publishing House, 1993.

Scalmer, Sean. *Gandhi in the West: The Mahatma and the Rise of Radical Protest.* Cambridge: Cambridge University Press, 2011.

Seier, Andrea. "Macht." In *Michel Foucault: Eine Einführung in sein Denken*, edited by Marcus S. Kleiner. Frankfurt am Main: Campus Verlag, 2001.

Singh, S. R. *History and Philosophy of Naturopathy.* Lucknow: Nature Cure Council of Medical Research, 1980.

UGLA. Sivasailam, Tamil Nadu. Accessed February 2016 <http://universalgoodlife.webs.com/>.

Smith-Morris, Carolyn. Introduction to *Diagnostic Controversy: Cultural Perspectives on Competing Knowledge in Healthcare*, edited by Carolyn Smith-Morris. New York: Routledge, 2016.

Solar Healing Center. Accessed February 2016 <http://solarhealing.com/>.

Som, Reba. Gandhi, Bose, Nehru and the Making of the Modern Indian Mind. New Delhi: Penguin, 2004.

Spitzer, Denise. "Ayurvedic Tourism in Kerala: Local Identities and Global Markets." In *Asia on Tour: Exploring the Rise of Asian Tourism*, edited by Tim Winter, Peggy Teo and T. C. Chang. Abingdon, Oxon: Routledge, 2009.

Sreedhara, Menon. *A Survey of Kerala History.* Madras: S. Viswanathan, 1991.

Srinivas, M. N. *Caste in Modern India and Other Essays.* Bombay: Asia Publishing House, 1962.

Street, Alice. "Artefacts of Not-Knowing: The Medical Record, Diagnosis and the Production of Uncertainty in Papua New Guinean Biomedicine." In *Social Studies of Science* 41, no. 6 (2011): 815-834.

Street, Alice. *Biomedicine in an Unstable Place: Infrastructure and Personhood in a Papua New Guinean Hospital.* London, Durham: Duke University Press, 2014.

Street, Alice and Simon Coleman. "Introduction: Real and Imagined Spaces." In *Space and Culture* 15, no. 1 (2012): 4-17.

Suhrud, Tridip. "Gandhi's Key Writings: In Search of Unity." In *The Cambridge Companion to Gandhi*, edited by Judith M. Brown and Anthony Parel. Cambridge: Cambridge University Press, 2011.

Sujatha, V. "Innovation within and between Traditions: Dilemma of Traditional Medicine in Contemporary India." In *Science, Technology and Society* 16, no. 2(2011): 191-213.

Sujatha, V. "The Patient as a Knower: Principle and Practice in Siddha Medicine." In *Economic and Political Weekly* 44, no. 16 (2009): 76-83.

Sujatha, V. "Pluralism in Indian Medicine: Medical Lore as a Genre of Medical Knowledge." In *Contributions to Indian Sociology* 41, no. 2 (2007): 169-202.

Sujatha, V. and Leena Abraham. Introduction to *Medical Pluralism in Contemporary India*, edited by V. Sujatha and Leena Abraham. Hyderabad: Orient Blackswan, 2012.

Sujatha, V. "Medicine State and Society: Indigenous Medicine and Medical Pluralism in India." In *Economic and Political Weekly* 44, no. 16 (2009): 35-43.

Sujeevitham. Cover picture, "How Biomedicine Killed Michael Jackson." P. B. No. 3055, Cochin, 682018 Kerala: Nature Life Hospital, October 2009.

Sujeevitham. Cover picture, "India, the Land of Pharma Drug Experiments." P. B. No. 3055, Cochin, 682018 Kerala: Nature Life Hospital, October 2008.

Sullivan, N. "Enacting Spaces of Inequality: Placing Global/State Governance within a Tanzanian Hospital." In *Space and Culture* 15, no. 1 (2012): 57-67.

Sunday Express Thailand. " A Natural Therapy for Children with HIV/AIDS is Tested at an Orphanage in Thailand." 2008.

Svoboda, Robert. "Theory and Practice of Ayurvedic Medicine." In *Oriental Medicine: An Illustrated Guide to the Asian Arts of Healing*, edited by Jan van Alphen and Anthony Aris. London: Serindia Publishing, 1995.

Swami Vivekananda Yoga Anusandhana Samsthana. Accessed February 2016 <http://www.svyasa.org/>.

Tamil Nadu Medical Dr. M.G.R. University. *Regulations for the Bachelor of Naturopathy and Yogic Sciences*. Unpublished Syllabus, available in the College. Chennai, 2005.

The Hindu. "CEE to allot 1525 MBBS seats, 19,470 engineering seats." Published December 6, 2009. Accessed February 2016 <http://www.thehindu.com/news/states/kerala/article60913.ece>.

Tirodkar, Manasi. "Cultural Loss and Remembrance in Contemporary Ayurvedic Medical Practice." In *Modern and Global Ayurveda: Pluralism and Paradigms*, edited by Dagmar Wujastyk and Frederick Smith. Albany: State University of New York Press, 2008.

Trawick, Margret. "An Ayurvedic Theory of Cancer." In *Medical Anthropology* 13, no. 1-2 (1991): 121-36.

Trivedi, Lisa: *Clothing Gandhi's Nation: Homespun and Modern India*. Bloomington: Indiana University Press, 2007.

Turner, Victor. "Variations on a Theme of Liminality." In *Secular Ritual*, edited by S. F. Moore and B. G. Myerhoff. Assen: Van Gorcum, 1977.

Uehleke, Bernhard and Hans-Dieter Hentschel. *Das große Kneipp-Gesundheitsbuch*. Stuttgart: Haug, 2006.

USA Today. "Yoga Copyright Raises Questions of Ownership." Published June 29, 2006. Accessed February 2016 <http://www.usatoday.com/money/2006-06-28-yoga-usat_x.htm>.

Vadakkanchery, Jacob. "CD1: A Bad Custom called Treatment," lecture, Nature Life Hospital, P. B. No. 3055, Cochin, 682018 Kerala, n. d., CD. Translated by Indu P.

Vadakkanchery, Jacob. "CD3: Allopathy- A Barbaric Treatment," lecture, Nature Life Hospital, P. B. No. 3055, Cochin, 682018 Kerala, n. d., CD. Translated by Indu P.

Vadakkanchery, Jacob. "CD 4: Can Poison be Medicine?", lecture, Nature Life Hospital, P. B. No. 3055, Cochin, 682018 Kerala, n. d., CD. Translated by Indu P.

Vadakkanchery, Jacob. "How Biomedicine Killed Michael Jackson." In *Sujeevitham,* October 2009. P. B. No. 3055, Cochin, 682018 Kerala: Nature Life Hospital, Oktober 2009.

Varma, C. R. R. "Difficulties in Treating Diseases," translated by Indu P. Payyanur: Varmaji Memorial Prakrithi Jeevana Trust, 2001a.

Varma, C. R. R.. "Health is a Truth, Disease is False. Devotion to Panchabotha and Ordinary Diseases," translated by Indu P. Payyanur: Varmaji Memorial Prakrithi Jeevana Trust, 2001b.

Varma, C. R. R.. "Kidney Diseases and Skin Diseases," translated by Indu P. Payyanur: Varmaji Memorial Prakrithi Jeevana Trust, 2001c.

Varma, Pavan K. *The Great Indian Middle Class.* New Delhi: Penguin, 1998.

Watters, Ethan: *Crazy Like Us: The Globalization of the American Psyche.* New York: Simon & Schusters, 2010.

Weiss, Mitchell G., Jayashree Ramakrishnab, and Daryl Sommac. "Health-Related Stigma: Rethinking Concepts and Interventions." In *Psychology, Health and Medicine* 11, no. 3 (2006): 227-87.

Weiss, Mitchell G., M. Isaac, S. R. Parkar, A. N. Chowdhury, and R. Raguram. "Global, National, and Local Approaches to Mental Health: Examples from India." *Tropical Medicine and International Health* 6, no. 1 (2001): 4–23.

Weiss, Richard S. *Recipes for Immortality: Medicine, Religion and Community in South India.* Oxford: Oxford University Press, 2009.

Wendel, Paul. *Standardized Naturopathy.* Brooklyn: Wendel, 1951.

Wettengl, Kurt. *Caspar David Friedrich: Winterlandschaften.* Leibzig: Seemann, 1990.

Wilson, Caroline. "The Commodification of Health Care in Kerala, South India: Science, Consumerism and Markets." PhD diss., University of Sussex, 2010b.

Wilson, Caroline. "'Eating, eating is always there': Food, Consumerism and Cardio-vascular Disease. Some Evidence from Kerala, South India." In *Anthropology and Medicine* 17, no. 3 (2010a): 261-75.

Wind, Gitte. "Negotiated Interactive Observation: Doing Fieldwork in Hospital Settings. In *Anthropology and Medicine* 15, no. 2 (2008): 79-89.

Wujastyk, Dagmar and Frederick M. Smith. *Modern and Global Ayurveda: Pluralism and Paradigms.* Albany: State University of New York Press, 2008.

Wujastyk, Dominik. *The Roots of Ayurveda.* London: Penguin, 2003.

Xavier, Denis , Prem Pais, P. J. Deveraux, Changchun Xie, D. Prabhakaran, and K. Srinath Reddy, and Rajeev Gupta, et al.: Treatment and Outcomes of Acute Coronary Syndromes in India (CREATE): A Prospective Analysis of Registry Data. In *Lancet* 371, no. 9622 (2008): 1435-42, 2008.

Young, Allen. "The Creation of Medical Knowledge: Some Problems in Interpretation." In *Social Science and Medicine* 15, no. 3 (1981): 379-86.

Young, Ken: "Consumption, Social Differentiation and Self-Definition of the New Rich in Industrialising Southeast Asia." In *Culture and Privilege in Capitalist Asia*, edited by Michael Pinches. London: Routledge, 1999.

Zaman, Shahaduz. *Broken Limbs, Broken Lives: Ethnography of a Hospital Ward in Bangladesh*. Amsterdam: Het Spinhuis, 2005.

Zaman, Shahaduz. "Poverty and Violence, Frustration and Inventiveness: Hospital Ward Life in Bangladesh." In *Social Science and Medicine* 59, no. 10 (2004): 2025-36.

Zimmermann, Francis. "The Scholar, the Wise Man, and Universals: Three Aspects of Ayurvedic Medicine." In *Knowledge and the Scholarly Medical Traditions*, edited by Don Bates. Cambridge: Cambridge University Press, 1995.

Zola, Irving. "Medicine as an Institution of Social Control." In *Sociological Review* 20, no. 4 (1972): 487-504.

Index